How to Lose 30 Pounds (Or More) In 30 Days With Juice Fasting

How To Lose Weight Fast, Keep it Off & Renew
The Mind, Body & Spirit Through Fasting,
Smart Eating & Practical Spirituality - Volume 3

ROBERT DAVE JOHNSTON

Published by:

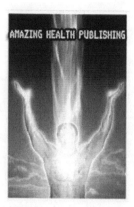

If you are interested in reading the next volume, follow Rob on Twitter @RobDaveJohnston

Copyright

Disclaimer & Legal Notices

The health-related information and suggestions contained in any of the books or written material mentioned above are based on the research, experience and opinions of the Author and other contributors. Nothing herein should be misinterpreted as actual medical advice, such as one would obtain from a Physician, or as advice for self-diagnosis or as any manner of prescription for self-treatment.

Neither is any information herein to be considered a particular or general cure for any ailment, disease or other health issue. The material contained within is offered strictly and solely for the purpose of providing Holistic health education to the general public. Persons with any health condition should consult a medical professional before entering this or any fasting, weight loss, detoxification or health related program.

Even if you suffer from no known illness, we recommend that you seek medical advice before starting any fasting, weight loss and/or detoxification program, and before choosing to follow any advice given this book. For any products or services mentioned or suggested in this book, you should read all packaging and instructions, as no substance, natural or drug, can be guaranteed to work in everyone.

Dedication

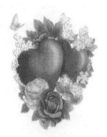

This series of books are dedicated to my mother Sonia Noemi, without whom I would not even be alive today. I love you mom. Thank you for never losing faith in me and supporting me, even when everything seemed hopeless and everyone else had given up on me. I owe you everything. I could collect all of the precious stones on this earth and lay them on your lap, and even still, I would not even come close to giving back to you all that you have given me.

Chapter 1
Fasting & The Holistic Revolution

Welcome to **How to Lose 30 Pounds (Or More) In 30 Days with Juice Fasting**. It takes a lot of courage to have purchased this book and actually be reading it now. Why? Because the fact that you are here means that you are willing to undergo a process of change.

A process that will be very rewarding but will present you with some challenges. I will make sure that these challenges serve to make you stronger, leaner and sharper. You are here, so you are willing to take the leap into the unknown, right? I am proud of you. But don't worry. I have gone through this road plenty of times. I will walk with you side-by-side and give you all of the information and motivation that you will need.

I am honored that you have purchased this book and placed your trust in me to give you quality information. And that is what you shall receive... for sure. Before we begin, there are a few things that I would like to share with you. Juice fasting has the power to transform your life. It can help you to lose massive amounts of weight quickly, as well as cleanse the body of disease-causing toxins that may have been hitching a ride in your vital organs for years. Even though fasting (*as a practice*) is rejected by traditional medicine, studies are coming to light which underscore its many health benefits. One of the most recent was a paper published **May 17, 2012 in Cell Metabolism**. In it, scientists from **Salk's Regulatory Biology Laboratory** found that: *"mice limited to eating during an 8-hour period are healthier than mice that eat freely throughout the day, regardless of the quality and content of their diet."* And there are others.

In April 2011, Utah-based Intermountain Medical Center revealed results of fasting research, indicating that, *"New evidence from cardiac researchers at the Intermountain Medical Center Heart Institute demonstrates that routine periodic fasting is also good for your health, and your heart. Research cardiologists are reporting that fasting not only lowers one's risk of coronary artery disease and diabetes, but also causes significant changes in a person's blood cholesterol levels.*

Both diabetes and elevated cholesterol are known risk factors for coronary heart disease. The discovery expands upon a 2007 Intermountain Healthcare study that revealed an association between fasting and reduced risk of coronary heart disease, the leading cause of death among men and women in America. In the new research, fasting was also found to reduce other cardiac risk factors, such as triglycerides, weight, and blood sugar levels."

Chapter 2
Fasting Scorned?

Did you see the amazing facts in that report? What do they do with these studies? Are they placed under a bird cage as garbage? **These are truly remarkable findings**. Why isn't the entire medical community raving about this and openly starting to promote fasting, or at least looking into it with more seriousness? Why is it that so many doctors dislike fasting so much when all evidence shows that, done properly, it could help prevent and possibly even cure many illnesses?

The above study, by itself, should be more than enough to start a huge mobilization of resources from the entire medical establishment. I'm not even saying that we have to drop everything and run to the hills barefoot shouting the praises of fasting. But, based on the research by Intermountain, *"ample evidence exists that, if given more attention (and respect) fasting could produce a variety of practical applications that would help many. The goal, in my mind, should be to bring fasting into the mainstream of preventive medicine."* Millions of people are sick and may die, and all along we have a powerful discipline that could help bring healing. Rather than using it to help mankind, the medical establishment prefers to shove it into a dark drawer, out of sight and mind like an ugly stepchild. Why? Instead of seizing the amazing promise that fasting presents, much of the medical community continues to squash the great promise that it holds. I am a layman who runs a website on fasting. Just a guy. Still, I can't tell you how many insulting messages I receive from doctors telling me that I am a traitor for promoting fasting and that I should go kill myself. Seriously, why is this? Have they not read the studies?

And it is my first-hand experience with fasting which gives me the certainty of the great ways it could be used to help others, particularly the obese and sick. Where were these doctors when I was dying of a liver condition and didn't have insurance? They certainly were not lining up to help me. No. But fasting saved my life and I want to pass that message to others. Fasting was always there for me. I did not need any insurance card to use it. And, in the same manner, fasting is here for you. There is, however, a rising movement that I hope will push holistic and preventive care to the forefront. The message is out there. Films like **Fat, Sick and Nearly Dead** and **Forks Over Knives** have done a great job at expanding public awareness about the amazing health benefits that fasting and holistic disciplines offer mankind. With the nation tangled in a web of dubious health care mandates, bitter political division, a rampant obesity epidemic and skyrocketing health care costs, what does the future hold? Indeed, right now it looks quite dim.

While politicians bicker and backbite one another as the country sinks further and further into insolvency, the time has come to seek for answers outside of the box. And alternative medicine is prepared to deliver... and deliver in a big way. The evidence is clear: *Fasting has the power to help millions of people dramatically improve the quality of their lives and health.*

Rather than continuing to medicate, the trend must be to educate ... let people know that assuming personal responsibility over lifestyle habits is the **doorway to tremendous breakthrough and national health revival**. I am sure that you know what I am talking about when I say 'personal responsibility.' Is that not what caused you to purchase this book and become willing to do the work? I guess my question is...

Who will stand and carry the message? At present, those who are suffering the most get gobbled up by a medical system that is always ready to cut, slice, dice, dissect and prescribe, but - as far as disease prevention goes, is stuck in the dark ages. **Individuals rising up and taking responsibility for their health is the key to this health revolution**. A revolution where holistic medicine can take its place beside the medical establishment and, together, they can join forces and resources to help make a real difference in the lives of millions.

Studies as the ones quoted above are helping to dispel negative preconceived notions about fasting and holistic medicine. And documentaries as the ones mentioned earlier are taking the message directly to the people, particularly as it relates to weight loss and health improvement.

All of these factors, combined, are creating an expanding informational centrifuge that, over time, will take our message to more and more people. And I predict that, within ten years, traditional and holistic medicine will begin to work side-by-side. As health care challenges continue to grow in complexity, what other choice do we really have? And the surge has already begun.

Colleagues in the holistic medicine industry have told me that over the past two years they've been seeing a marked surge in the number of new patients. I am not a doctor, but I agree with their assessment. My own website, **FitnessThroughFasting.com**, has been around for almost seven years. Traffic has notably spiked in the past year as awareness increases of the benefits of fasting. Colleagues who run websites similar to mine also report a rise in web visitors.

I hope against hope that, someway somehow, old prejudices against fasting and holistic medicine (*from doctors as well as the general public*) will erode as more evidence mounts about the awesome healing power that the fasting discipline wields. And today, YOU will become one of the believers as you experience the quick weight loss and cleansing that juice fasting always provides.

Chapter 3
Fasting & Weight Loss

To give you a better idea of the work we will carry out in this book, let's take a look at the various kinds of fasting practices and the approximate weight loss .they produce.

Water Fasting is considered the purest form of fasting and involves exactly that: **going a period of time without eating and drinking only water.** Weight loss while water fasting usually ranges from 1 to 20 pounds (*or more*) in the first seven days. After that, the body (*commonly*) settles into a fat-burning '*pace*' of **one-to-three pounds per day**.

Specific weight loss figures will depend on how the body responds, as well as a person's overall state of health.   Twenty to 30% of the initial weight lost with water fasting is water weight, not fat. Once the longer-term pace is reached, water weight loss diminishes. At that point the body will '*eat*' one-to-three pounds of pure fat daily. Again, these numbers fluctuate according to a person's body makeup and general health.

Absolute Fasting. (*also known as dry fasting*) is the hardest and strictest form of fasting. It entails going a period of time (*no more than 72 hours are recommended*) without eating **OR** drinking liquids of any kind. There are two kinds of absolute fasting: *soft and dry*. Soft dry fasting allows '*external*' contact with water as taking a shower, going swimming etc. With <u>hard</u> dry fasting, the practitioner abstains from **ALL** contact with water, even showering.

Dry fasting produces the fastest and most dramatic weight loss, approximately 20 pounds in three days. Most of the weight loss, however, is comprised of water weight because the body goes into dehydration. Although there aren't many studies about dry fasting, it is often used by bodybuilders during a competition to maximize muscle definition.

There are some who maintain that absolute fasting could cure the common cold if practiced when symptoms first emerge. I have read cases of people who have done an absolute fast for three-to-five days and were reportedly cured of life-long allergic reactions and conditions. The process behind the healing power of dry fasting is that, since the body is not receiving food or hydration, overall body functions slow down to a minimum. Consequently, it is believed, the immune system has a much greater amount of resources to seek and destroy all sort of sickness - even viruses.

While with juice and water fasting bodily functions slow down considerably, a dry fast reduces them much further. This deeper reduction in body functions, it is believed, gives the immune system ultra-healing capacity. Sort of like having been stuck in a traffic jam and then, suddenly, having the entire interstate all to yourself. You don't have to share the highway any longer.

Therefore, you can step on the gas pedal freely because the traffic with which you were sharing the road is no longer there. I complctcd a 72-hour dry fast some years ago and can tell you that it is probably among the hardest things I've ever done. You can read more about my dry fasting experience at the main website **FitnessThroughFasting.com**. Dry fasting is dangerous and should not be practiced unless one is **<u>VERY</u>** experienced in fasting and calorie restriction.

<u>Juice Fasting</u>. is the most popular kind of fasting and the one we will practice in this book. .Juice fasting is a time during which one ingests only water as well as the juice from liquefied fruits and vegetables. Juice fasting is popular because it is not as harsh as water or dry fasting. Rather than relying only on water, it pumps the body full of amazing nutrients. We will look in detail at the amazing health-giving benefits of fruits and vegetables in a later chapter. Overall, weight loss with juice fasting in the first 10 days can fluctuate from 7 to 20 pounds (*depending on health and body makeup*), and then settles on one-to-two pounds per day.

That is why the title of this book is "**How to Lose 30 Pounds (Or More) In 30 Days With Juice Fasting.**" Personal experience (*and through helping others*) has shown me time and time again that 30 days of juice fasting <u>can easily lead to weight loss of 30 pounds or more</u>. That is a very short time in which to lose such a large amount of weight. One (*obese*) gentleman I worked with some years ago actually lost 75 pounds during a 30-day juice fast.

If you follow my instructions, you too will lose a huge amount of weight in only 30 days. That's what makes juice fasting so awesome. It produces supersonic weight loss while still allowing you to feed on powerful nutrients. Most of us do not have the luxury of *'dropping everything'* and taking a 30-day vacation; so juicing becomes the **most feasible way to practice this discipline -> without completely eliminating food intake.**

In this book, I will give you all of the information and motivation that you'll need to launch a 30-day juice fast and lose 30 pounds or more. In addition to the rapid weight loss, you will also revolutionize your health. Juice fasting is one of the most powerful and amazing healing sources available to man. Juice Fasting has been known to help the body fight-off severe and chronic illnesses. I cannot guarantee that you will be healed if you are sick. I CAN, however, tell you that juice fasting is one of the best gifts you can give your body. With juice fasting, you will place your body in an excellent position to receive a tremendous jolt of health and nutrition. Many have been healed with juice fasting. There is no reason why the same cannot happen to you.

Chapter 4
How Fasting Works

Here I want to talk briefly about the process that fasting kicks into motion, and how the body respond when calories are restricted. The amazing process that I am referring to is known as **ketosis**.

Ketosis is the term used to describe the body's response to calorie-restriction. When in ketosis, the body stops acquiring its energy resources from food and begins to 'eat' stored fat as fuel. Ketosis usually starts after 10-to-16 hours of abstaining from food. It may induce a *'flu-like'* sickness known as a Curative or Healing Crisis . We will look at detox symptoms in the 'motivational messages' part of the book. The healing crisis is put into motion as the body begins to tap into stored fat for food, causing large amount of accumulated toxins to be released into the bloodstream.

This is similar to being vaccinated. If you have received a vaccine, you know that hours later one tends to start feeling a bit under the weather. The reason is that the vaccine fills the body with disease-causing microorganisms and a temporary sickness ensues. The same happens when the body goes into ketosis. Toxins stored within fat cells are suddenly let loose to roam freely. Temporary intoxication results - the curative crisis. Through this process, the body works very hard to expel the toxins through the skin (*perspiration*), urine and feces. Ketosis continues until the fast is broken as the body continues to devour stored fat for fuel. The healing crisis, however, typically ends after 9-to-14 days, indicating that the body has processed and eliminated all of the toxins. At this time one usually starts to feel stronger and more alert. The healing crisis vanishes and you will likely feel little or no hunger. Many people tell me that, once they reach this phase, they feel that they can go on fasting indefinitely. To be sure, this is the most pleasant part of the fast. It is like fighting the fierce fire in the atmosphere and then finally breaking through and entering outer space. That 'outer space' experience, I believe, is what ultimate health is all about. It is the condition that we are all entitled to attain, IF we are willing to pay the price. And I believe that you ARE willing to pay the price. Otherwise you wouldn't have bought this book, right?

How Long Can One Fast?

Most (*healthy and average-sized*) individuals can usually <u>water fast</u> for as long as 40 days before the onset of '<u>real</u>' starvation. By the time the healing crisis ends, hunger pangs are reduced and (*in most cases*) become but a minor irritation. Hunger then returns (*with a vengeance*) at around day 40 of water fasting (or more depending on each person's body fat levels). The return of hunger (the second hunger as it is referred to) indicates that the body has consumed all of the stored fat and has now begun to feed on live tissue. This is the start of real starvation. The fast **MUST** be broken at once. I experienced this '*second hunger*' years ago when I first started to practice water fasting.

It was a very scary experience as I literally felt my skin and muscles being chewed from the inside out. That was my own carelessness. Fasting should <u>never</u> get to that phase. With juice fasting, one can typically go indefinitely so long as the juice is made properly. I did a 100-day juice fast years ago and it was a very rewarding experience. I did not do it for weight loss per se, yet ended up losing 105 pounds. A juice fast of this length should include some protein via the mixture of crushed nuts, oils, tofu or <u>spirulina</u>, the amazing micro salt water plant that contains rich vegetable protein, even more than meat or fish. If a long juice fast includes these additional (and necessary) ingredients, one could possibly continue juice fasting indefinitely. This, however, is not common. The longest juice fasts that are normally carried out range from 30 to 60 days. And, honestly... 30 days of juice fasting is more than enough to start. You can always fast again later for a longer period of time once you get used to the practice and get to know how your body responds with long-term calorie restriction.

Eating After Fasting

Still, **it is important for me to emphasize**: While fasting is wonderful and the results can be tremendous, it is **NOT** the fasting in itself that makes the difference. Rather, it is what you decide to do **AFTER** the fast which will determine the **TRUE** benefits that you will receive. Fasting for a hundred days only to return to eating poorly is a cop-out and not at all what I want to teach you. I get tons of emails from people wanting to learn about what happens with 40, 60 ... 90-day juice and water fasts. They are interested in quick weight loss, which is fine. However, when I ask them what they intend to do once the fast is over, I either not hear from them again or get a very vague answer like, "*I'll eat better.*" That type of anemic response tells me that the person has thought a great deal about weight loss, but very little about what he or she intends to do to keep the weight off when the fast is over. **So my message to you is this**: If you are truly serious about losing weight and keeping it off, it is imperative that you realize that **PERMANENT** eating-habit changes are necessary for long-term success.

You can lose 30 pounds or more through our work together. But if you do nothing more... if you have not planned ahead as to what your diet will be when the fast ends, then you are setting yourself up for failure. **Let me be blunt**: *Nothing sucks as bad as fasting for 30 days, going through the hunger, detox and sacrifice to lose weight, only to see yourself balloon right back up in a few short weeks after the fast because you didn't change your eating habits*. And I can <u>guarantee you</u> that, if you do not change your eating habits, then chances are **VERY** high that you **WILL** regain the weight you lose by fasting within three months. I need you to be very aware of this reality now when we are just getting started. Ponder on what I've just said as we move forward. At the end of the book I will give you suggestions on meal structures that you may want to adopt for good. However, **YOU** are the one that has to be convinced.

Here's the bottom line: fasting for weight loss <u>without</u> a plan for permanent eating-habit changes is a waste of time and will **<u>NOT</u>** produce the long-term success that you desire. Lucky for you, you have me in your corner and I will be nagging the daylights out of you all through this book until you get the message! My goodness... am I raving? :-)

Chapter 5
Items You Will Need

To successfully complete our work, there are some key pieces of hardware that you will need - **primarily a juicer and a blender**. If you do not own this hardware, then it is important for you to purchase the items before moving forward. Blenders are very cheap. You can probably find a good one for around $20. You may even find one in your home's storage room at the bottom shelf next to the Neil Sedaka 8-track tapes. What I mean is that most houses have a blender 'somewhere,' so take a good look around before you go out and buy one.

As far as juicers, you can find them as cheap as $40-$50 and as expensive as $400-$500. My suggestion is that you purchase the best one that your budget allows. This juicer will be taking quite a beating. You will be running it at full power for at least half an hour every three-to-four days. That is six times weekly and more than 24 times in 30 days. The juicer will be crushing soft produce as tomatoes and strawberries, as well as harder ones like broccoli and cauliflower stems. **What I'm trying to say is this:** The juicer we need has to be good. I remember some time ago I was out of town and fasting for 21 days. I purchased the cheapest juicer in the store and, lo' and behold', it lasted two days. I don't want your juicing efforts to be interrupted by broken hardware. **Get the very best one that you can**.

Consider the juicer an investment in your health and future. If you have to not buy some other things in order to purchase it, then so be it. Ok? I'm not saying that you should go in debt to buy a juicer. Just buy the very best one that you can and, if need be, consider stretching your budget a little to get a solid and lasting model. I could write volumes upon volumes describing the different kinds of juicers available in the market. To keep it simple, I will give you some of my personal favorites.

Juicer Recommendations

I have tried nearly every juicer under the sun. I use them without mercy, I pound them, I shove hard stems in the feeder and force the blades to work overtime. I go to town with these juicers... no mercy. Based on this experience *(over the past 15 years)*, I can safely recommend the **Breville Fountain Juicer** which costs $180 at Amazon.com. The Breville is my favorite. It takes my beatings and keeps on grinning. Another good one is the **Jack Lalane JLPJB**. It is also available at Amazon.com and costs $100. Any of these two will get the job done very nicely. An interesting model that I tested recently is the **Jay Kordich JDJB21001 Deluxe 2-in-1 Juicer and Blender**. I like the whole juicer/blender combination idea. I used it for around one week and it took all of my abuse and produced good juice. The blender part of the unit works well and will fill the bill in our case. At $89 *(amazon.com)*, the **Jay Kordich** is a good piece of hardware.

You may wish to visit your local discount store. There are always good deals on juicers. You may be able to find a good one for $40 to $50. Whatever you do, stay away from **Juiceman** juicers. They totally blow. I owned three and they all crapped out on me within the first month of ownership. Steer clear.

Good juicer brands are Cuisinart, Hamilton Beach, Oster and... maybe Black and Decker. I say Black & Decker guardedly because I've had some bitter moments operating those juicers. Whatever you decide to buy, the investment will be well worth it. I want juicing to become a **<u>PERMANENT</u>** part of your lifestyle, so I hope that these appliances will be used regularly in your home well after this fast has ended.

Chapter 6
How to Use This Book

Let me explain how all of this is going to work. Since there is **A LOT** of information I want to share with you, this book is structured to take you in a linear direction towards the start of your fast, working through each of the 30 days and then breaking the fast. **HOWEVER**, that does not mean that you **HAVE TO** juice fast for 30 days straight in order to receive benefit. There are a variety of intermittent alternatives that you also can consider if you think that 30 days may be too much for you right now. That is fine. I understand. You can start slow and work your way towards it.

In between, you will gain a lot of inner strength and understanding of how your body works. Whether you want to do 30 days of uninterrupted juice fasting, or if you want to start but do not wish to go that far at this time, this book can help you get there. I have thrown the kitchen's sink into this book so that you can have a step-by-step program that you can follow without confusion. In the next chapter we will start picking up speed by looking in detail at the **health benefits and nutrients in fruits and vegetables**. I want you to fully-internalize the powerful boost that you will be giving your body, and I will list many of the **health conditions that each of the fruits and vegetables are known to fight (and help heal)**. Yeah, this is the part that has a lot of nutrient names that are hard to spell, let alone pronounce.

But, please... go through the material with me. This is all put together for **YOU.** It is all for **YOUR** benefit. If you give it a chance, I think you will be amazed at the **incredible, tremendous and totally earth-shattering nutrients and disease-fighting properties that fruits and vegetables have**. I get very excited each time I read about it. I don't have to rely only on doctors or medications. I can take my juicer, a bowl of fruits and vegetables, and I am basically injecting my body with pure life - beyond anything that can be described or fathomed.

To Clarify: I'm not saying that I do **NOT** go see a doctor if I need to or take medications if I must. I do. I believe in traditional medicine. I think it has slanted way too much towards treating disease rather than preventing. However, I still do what I have to do to take care of my body. What I mean is that, in addition to doctors and any medications, I like to push the envelope and do **everything that I can for my health**. And juice fasting is what brings it all together for me.

Once we look at the nutrients in fruits and vegetables, and the diseases that they are known to protect against (*and even cure*), I will give you a *'basic recipe'* of fruits and vegetables that you can use to do the fast. If you are new to juice fasting, this basic recipe will be very helpful because you won't have to *'guess'* which fruits and vegetables to use. If you are experienced, you can experiment as much as you wish or use your favorite recipe. For the sake of simplicity, however, the basic recipe is a combination that I've used for many years. It is very powerful and will help you get started quickly. I will give you a weekly shopping list of the fruits and vegetables that you'll need to prepare. From there we will move on to detailed instructions on how to use the juicer, how to prepare the fruits and vegetables for juicing, how to actually juice the produce, how to store it and how much to drink each day that you are fasting. You will then pick a date to start the fast. I will give you a **FIVE-STEP** structure you can use to build a strong support and motivational foundation. Once you begin the fast, you will have my **TOP TEN** motivational messages to **read and reflect on as you move through the fast**. The messages have been written from my own fasting experiences and are there to **help you cross through hunger, detox symptoms and the other mental challenges that arise while fasting**. The messages will provide instructions to help make the fast as easy as possible. I strongly suggest that you follow those instructions as they are based on many years of *'trial and error,'* so I know that they work.

THEN, I will give you detailed instructions on how to break the fast, as well as dietary recommendations for you to consider adopting in perpetuity. As I told you before, breaking a fast is the **MOST IMPORTANT** part of the process because the choices you make **THEN** will determine whether you adopt new eating habits or return to the old way of things. If you return to poor eating, then the weight loss and health benefits will be short-lived.

If, on the other hand, you make a decision to **PERMANENTLY CHANGE YOUR EATING HABITS** (*as I hope you do*), then you can expect to enjoy the weight loss and health benefits for <u>many years to come</u>. I know that I said this before. However, I cannot emphasize just how important the post-fast phase is. To that end, I have also written a much more detailed book called "**How to (Properly) Break a Fast and Keep The Weight Off**" which I suggest you read as well. It goes a lot deeper into this crucial *'post-fasting'* process.

So there's our plan. Yes, it's **<u>A LOT</u>** of material. But, don't worry. Let's just take it step-by-step. A little bit at a time, we will make it through. Stick with me and let me guide you through. You aren't alone. I am here with you all the way!

Chapter 7
Be Persistent & Realistic

I always like to say: Rome was not built in a day, but it **WAS** built! No matter what your weight loss and health-improvement goals may be, juice fasting can help you get there. I know that because **I have experienced it for myself**. I suffered from a severe liver illness years ago when I first started fasting. I was dying... literally. I spent more than 20 years trapped in the hell off binge eating disorder, losing my body, my mind... my soul. Today, the illness is still in my body, but it is nearly dormant and is no longer life-threatening. People ask me why I'm not bitter that others get healed and yet I still have the sickness in my body, albeit inactive.

I have nothing but gratitude in my heart. I really should be dead. And what is left of the illness in my body, I believe, is there to 'remind me' from whence I came. A friend of mine always says: "Those who tend to forget, tend to repeat." And I never want to repeat that misery again. So I am thankful. Juice fasting has changed my perspective on health and personal responsibility. I have been persistent with "*the process*" and allowed time to pass. Most important of all, I no longer eat the garbage that I used to. I exercise and fast regularly. I have matured emotionally and spiritually. **All of this has taught me to make better choices for myself**. You see what I am saying? **DO NOT** fixate your mind on that things have to happen **ONLY A CERTAIN WAY**. That unless you lose ALL of the weight in one shot on your first attempt, that fasting doesn't work. It took some attempts before I finally achieved my breakthrough. So this book is not written as a *'miracle cure'* or *'overnight success'* manual. Yes, juice fasting will help you to lose a lot of weight in a short period of time. But more than just fasting is needed. You must put all of your energy into this task. Open your heart and mind to what comes.

As I said before, if you are unable to do the entire 30 days of juice fasting at this time, shoot for three days... work your way up from there a little bit at a time. This is not a race. Rather, it is a marathon... you can pace yourself at the beginning, work your way through the rough spots and accelerate later when you feel more confident. There is no **WRONG** to practice juice fasting. What matters is that you get in the saddle and start working at it. Even 24 hours once a week for starters is terrific. And <u>NEVER</u> put yourself down if you fall short and stumble. Whether you reach your goals right away or it takes a little bit of time, you **WILL** reach them if you stick to it and practice. **No matter what, no matter what, no matter what... DO NOT allow bitterness, unbelief and/or self-pity to stop you**. This is just the beginning of a whole new life for you.

I think the **Spirit of The Universe** sometimes gives us a fishing rod rather than drop the '<u>fish</u>' in our laps. In other words, if everything is easy and immediate, what have I really learned? In which way have I grown as a human being? What is to keep me from returning to the behavior that caused the situation in the first place? On the other hand if, through some trial and error, I am given the "*character*" to change and produce a better life, **THEN** I can hang on to the results that I achieve **FOR LIFE**. In season or out of season, <u>you will know what to do and what not to do</u> because, through persistence and heart, **the miracle has happened in your mind, belief systems and behavior**. Now **THAT** is a **TRUE** miracle, don't you think?

Reminder: This book has instructions for a "*long-term*" or extended fast. Fasting for more than 2 days should be done with caution and respect. If you are unsure about the state of your health, I urge you to see your doctor <u>before</u> you continue. This book focuses on fasting for weight loss & health betterment – **NOT** for ascetic purposes. Fasting for a season to lose excess weight and get healthier is acceptable. **Abuse of it via Anorexic and Bulimic practices is NOT** . If you have struggled with an eating disorder, I urge you to set this book aside and seek help before you consider any type of calorie restriction. Ok, let's jump right into the amazing power of fruits and vegetables!

Chapter 8
Pork, Toothpicks & Diet Sodas

I am sure you probably have heard how important it is to *"eat your fruits and vegetables."* Yes, I heard it a lot when I was growing up. My grandmother was adamant about it! Unfortunately, I always preferred candy and pastries – anything sweet. My grandfather used to run a candy and finger-food store out of the house. Kids would come in through the kitchen window and order sodas, candy and all types of goodies. The smell of fried foods always filled the house. The scent of food was my drug... it got me high. It just took over all of my senses and made me obsessed with eating.

At night, I would wake up when everyone was asleep and raid the candy store. When my grandmother would come to my room to sweep and clean up, she would find countless candy wrappers under the bed. "You are eating all of our profits Rob," she would say with a half-smile and both hands on her waist. And that wasn't all. When I was around 7 or 9, my grandmother and mother owned a clothing store. It was located in a shopping mall. In the back of the mall was a man in a hot dog cart selling pig skin and other ridiculously-fattening food. I would walk over to the cart and buy the biggest plate available. The man would serve my overflowing plate and cover it with another plate on top. He would give me a set of toothpicks to eat as most of it was finger food.

Then I would start walking back towards the clothing store, all the while grease sliding down my clothes and onto the ground. That walk from the cart to the store, to me, was like a heroin addict who had just bought his fix and was walking towards the place where he could get high. The sense of desperation was always there as I walked towards the store. The smell of the fat made me crazy.

By the time I got to the store, I was literally salivating like a dog. I would walk into the store, ignore everyone around me and walk straight to the storage room in the back of the store. I would close the door behind me, sit down on a bench that was there, place the plate on a table, grab the toothpicks and start eating and eating and eating like a slob as the grease covered my clothes from top to bottom. Oh, and along with the junk food I would always buy a *'Diet Coke.'* My grandma would look at me and laugh. *"That is some diet Robert,"* she would say. They saw me as just a young boy with a big appetite. But the sickness was already festering inside of me. And so, that behavior marked my childhood, part of my teenage years and many of my adult years. Today I have learned – *through much pain and failure* - that I had to admit that **my way just wasn't working.** I had to find a better way to live or I was going to die. Why did I tell you this whole sob story? Because I want you to know that I made it out from that condition and have reached my goals. I am sure that you have stories of your own.

If you have been overweight for a long time, then it is likely that there are some similarities between your store and mine. At the very least, we are comrades in the road to self-mastery. We both want to overcome all habits and behaviors that lead us to become unhealthy and overweight, right? And, as comrades in the journey, we now come together to enter into the solution. Grandma was right. Fruits and vegetables are still the answer! And, as I have come to realize, juicing on a regular basis totally fulfills this important (*and healthy*) objective. It keeps me clean, lean and very grateful to have overcome all of those dark years of binging, obesity and food addiction.

So let's move forward and get to know the nutrients in our fruits and vegetables. Let's see what each of these have to offer you at this phase in your life.

Chapter 9
Nutrition in Colors

The popular phrase *"eating a rainbow"* is an easy way to remember that color variety when juicing is where the real power is. Variety is the best way to give your body the broadest range possible of vital nutrients. Let us take a look at each color category of fruits and vegetables and the ways in which they can each protect and heal our bodies.

Red Fruits & Vegetables

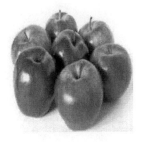

Contain nutrients such as lycopene, ellagic acid, Quercetin, and Hesperidin, to name a few. These nutrients lessen the risk of prostate cancer, lower blood pressure, help reduce tumor growth and LDL cholesterol levels, hunt harmful free-radicals, and ease arthritis.

Orange & Yellow

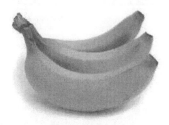

Contain beta-carotene, zeaxanthin, flavonoids, lycopene, potassium, and vitamin C.

These nutrients can reduce age-related macular degeneration, the risk of prostate cancer, and LDL cholesterol.

They also help control blood pressure, support collagen formation, fight harmful free radicals, regulate acid/base balance, and aid in building healthy bones.

Green Vegetables

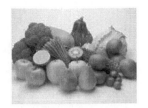

Green vegetables contain, most importantly, chlorophyll. They also contain large amounts of fiber, lutein, zeaxanthin, calcium, folate, vitamin C, and Beta-carotene.

The nutrients found in these vegetables decrease cancer risks, help control blood pressure and increase HDL (*the "good" cholesterol*) levels.

They normalize digestion, support healthy vision, fight harmful free-radicals, and boost the immune system.

Blue & Purple

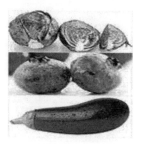

Contain nutrients which include lutein, zeaxanthin, resveratol (*has powerful anti-aging properties*) vitamin C, fiber, flavonoids, ellagic acid, and quercetin.

Similar to the other vegetable colors, these support retinal health, lower LDL cholesterol, boost the immune system, support healthy digestion, improve calcium and other mineral absorption, and reduce inflammation, tumor growth and carcinogens in the body.

White

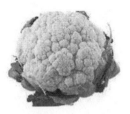

Contain nutrients such as beta-glucans, EGCG, SDG, and lignans that provide powerful immune boosting activity.

These nutrients also balance hormone levels and strengthen the body's disease-killing B and T cells, thus reducing the risk of colon, breast, and prostate cancers.

Chapter 10
Detoxify & Heal

As you can see, each fruit and vegetable color has distinctive nutrients that are essential to the human body. These nutrients have the power to detoxify the body and, in many cases heal disease. I totally believe that my binge eating disorder and food addictions were cured by these very nutrients we are talking about. Fruits and vegetables are "*whole*" foods, created by nature. The processed foods that most people eat **CANNOT** compare to the life-giving power of – *say* - strawberries or broccoli, which contain crucial fiber, vitamins, and enzymes.

To give you a specific point of reference, I put together a chart of fruits and vegetables divided into their respective color category. You will now have a very comprehensive view of the huge power that juice fasting has to offer you. I am giving you all of this information in hopes that, long after the fast is over, you will adopt juicing as a permanent part of your lifestyle I **STRONGLY** recommend that you experiment with this chart and find a combination you like and can prepare on your own once the fast is over. Here you have a mighty tool that will help you become a proficient juicing practitioner. **The chart below is like receiving a map to a new and mysterious world**. It looks very exciting on paper, but it is up to you to decide which continent you wish to explore. You have to plan your journey and then actually start it.

Do not let apathy and/or laziness keep you from launching your expedition. Believe me, it is well worth it and can literally alter the course of your life, as it did mine. If you are new to juicing, don't worry. Simply follow the basic recipe I will outline and you will be on your way. You can experiment with the chart later once you feel more comfortable with the process.

Veggie Chart (By Color)

Green	White	Red	Yellow/Orange	Blue/Purple
Artichokes	Brown pears	Beets	Apricots	Black Currants
Arugula	Cauliflower	Blood oranges	Bananas	Black Salsify
Asparagus	Dates	Cherries	Butternut	Blackberries
Avocados	Garlic	Cranberries	Squash	Blueberries
Broccoflower	Ginger	Guava	Cantaloupe	Dried plums
Broccoli	Jerusalem	Papaya	Cape	Eggplant
Broccoli Rabe	Artichoke	Pink Grapefruit	Gooseberries	Elderberries
Brussel	Jicama	Pink/Red	Carrots	Grapes
sprouts	Kohlrabi	grapefruit	Golden Kiwifruit	Plums
Celery	Mushrooms	Pomegranates	Grapefruit	Pomegranates
Chayote	Onions	Radicchio	Lemon	Prunes
Squash	Parsnips	Radishes	Mangoes	Purple Belgian
Chinese	Potatoes	Raspberries	Nectarines	endive
cabbage	Shallots	Red apples	Oranges	Purple Potatoes
Cucumbers	Turnips	Red bell	Papayas	Purple
Endive	White Corn	peppers	Peaches	Asparagus
Green apples	White	Red chili	Persimmons	Purple cabbage
Green beans	Nectarines	Peppers	Pineapples	Purple carrots
Green	White	Red grapes	Pumpkin	Purple figs
Cabbage	Peaches	Red onions	Rutabagas	Purple grapes
Green grapes		Red pears	Sweet corn	Purple peppers
Green onion		Red peppers	Sweet potatoes	Raisins
Green pears		Red potatoes	Tangerines	
Green		Rhubarb	Yellow apples	
Peppers		Strawberries	Yellow beets	
Honeydew		Tomatoes	Yellow figs	
Kiwifruit		Watermelon	Yellow pears	
Leafy greens			Yellow peppers	
Leeks			Yellow Potatoes	
Lettuce			Yellow summer	
Limes			Squash	
Okra			Yellow	
Peas			Tomatoes	
Sno Peas			Yellow	
Spinach			Watermelon	
Sugar snap			Yellow winter	
Peas			Squash	
Watercress				
Zucchini				

Chapter 11
Key Nutrients

To get the message across with greater force, let us take one more glance at the amazing nutrients that juicing places at your disposal.

Quercetin, which is found in apples, onions and other citrus fruits. It not only prevents LDL cholesterol oxidation, but also helps the body cope with allergens and other lung and breathing problems.

Ellagic Acid, which is mainly found in raspberries, strawberries, pomegranates, and walnuts, has been proven in many clinical studies to act as an antioxidant and anti-carcinogen in the gastrointestinal tract. This nutrient also has been proven to have an anti-proliferative effect on cancer cells, because it decreases their ATP production.

Carotenoids – the best known is beta-carotene, which is converted into vitamin A upon entering the liver. Although being widely known for its positive effects on eyesight, it has also been proven to decrease LDL cholesterol levels.

Lycopene is mainly found in tomatoes and has been found to decrease the risk of prostate cancer, as well as protect against heart disease. Especially for men over 40 years of age, this nutrient is of great importance.

Lutein, which is found in blueberries and members of the squash family, is important for healthy eyes. However, it does support your heart too, helping to prevent against coronary artery disease.

Flavonoids, which include anthocyanins, flavones, isoflavones, proantocyanidins, quercetin and more, are found almost everywhere. Flavonoids are responsible for the colors in the skins of fruits and vegetables and help to stop the growth of tumor cells and are potent antioxidants. They also can reduce inflammation.

Beta-Glucan, found in mushrooms, stabilizes and balances the body's immune system by supporting white blood cells. EGCG, which can be found in tea, has been shown to reduce the risk of colon and breast cancer. It boosts the immune system and encourages T-cell formation, which defends our body against sickness and disease.

Bioflavonoids, which are found in citrus fruits, are considered a companion to vitamin C because they strengthen the action of that vitamin in the body. These nutrients also help to lower cholesterol levels and support collagen in the joints.

Vitamin C is scattered throughout the spectrum of fruits, but is most commonly associated with oranges and other citrus fruits. Potassium, which is a nutrient many Americans are deficient in, is absolutely essential for the heart and circulatory system.

Another good food component many people don't get enough of is **fiber**, found in fruits, vegetables, and whole grains. If you suffer from constipation or various forms of digestive system distress as Acid Reflux or Crohn's Disease, juice fasting can go a long ways in helping the body heal.

Wow, that is all pretty amazing. There must be something to that *"eat your fruits and veggies"* thing my grandma always said. Are you able to see the power of what you are about to do? Do you see why this moment in your life is so important? If you have practiced juice fasting before, then you know the immense power that is behind a 30-day juice fast with this powerhouse of nutrients. Take it in and rejoice. Your life is going to change my friend. The potency of what you are about to do is beyond description!

Chapter 12
Basic Juicing Recipe

Now let's look at the shopping list that you will need to fill to successfully complete your 30-day fast. **Note**: It is preferable, if you can afford it, that you purchase organic fruits and vegetables. Organic does not have the pesticides that are used to grow most of the produce in our supermarkets. If this is beyond your current budget, then it is vital that you spend some time thoroughly washing each fruit and vegetable **BEFORE** starting the juicing process – which I will walk you through at a later chapter.

Shopping List

Below are the fruits and veggies that you will need. Some of them will need to be purchased **WEEKLY.** Every three days (*more or less*) you will prepare **ONE GALLON** of juice. This gallon will be consumed over a three-day period. In other words, each batch of fruits and veggies that you purchase will allow you to make around 2.5 gallons of juice. And you will be drinking anywhere from 48 to 64 ounces of juice daily.

Therefore, each trip to the market should yield enough juice for seven days of fasting. I will talk more about portions later, but these figures should give you a general idea of what we are striving towards.

Here's the shopping list:

* 2 Packages of Celery
* 5 Medium-to-Large Tomatoes
* 1 Full Head of Broccoli
* 1 Bag of Large Carrots (*not the mini ones*)
* 1 Heaping Handful of Watercress
* 1 Large Chunk of Pumpkin
* 6 Apples (*cheaper if bought by the bag*)
* 1 Basket of Blueberries
* 1 Basket of Strawberries
* 1 Bag of Oranges
* 5 Lemons
* 4 Bananas
*1 Bottle of Vegetable Juice (*V-8 is fine. Low sodium preferable*)
* 2 Large & Deep Bowls (*Tupperware is fine*)
* 1 Half-Gallon Plastic Jug With a Tight Lid
* 1 Gallon Plastic Jug With a Tight Lid
* 1 Roll of Aluminum Foil
* 1 Cutting Board
* 1 Sharp Knife to Cut and Peel
* 2 Six-Packs of Seltzer Water (*Sparkling Water, Club Soda*)
* 1 Box of Decaffeinated Green Tea (*You may need to go to a health food store to find this decaf type*)
* 1 Box of Chamomile Tea
* Tryptophan Amino Acid 500mg Tablets (*To help you sleep in case of insomnia and to help stabilize mood*)
* Valerian Root Capsules (*To help calm and settle you down, particularly at night*)
* One 24-Pack of Bottled Water (*Get it even if you have a reliable water filter. If you go out, you want to have a few with you*)
*1 Ice Cooler (*if you spend a lot of time out of the home. carry some juice with you*)

And, of course, we also need the **blender and juicer as mentioned at the start of this book**. That's pretty much it. Some of the produce you will only need to get once or twice as, for example, oranges and apples which can be kept refrigerated for longer periods of time without spoiling. After the first two times of preparing the juice, you will have a better idea of the exact quantities that you need. You may need more... you may need less. The quantities I have given you are based on a general average of what will be needed.

Make sure that the bowls are big enough to hold all of the produce diced and peeled. So I would suggest that you err in the side of caution and get two big ones. The same goes with the cutting board. Get a larger one just to be sure that you can cut comfortably without scratching your kitchen counter. Moreover, I have asked you to get both a 1/2 gallon and a 1 gallon jug. The reason is that if you go out during the day, you can use the smaller jug to carry some juice.

The rest of the juice can be kept refrigerated at home and covered in aluminum foil. The juice is powerful but delicate. It is a good idea to cover the jug with foil to protect the juice from light. These jugs <u>must</u> have tight lids that won't easily open. You definitely do <u>NOT</u> want to spill and waste any of the juice! The ice cooler has always been my best friend because I drive a lot and always keep it in the back seat packed with ice, drinking water, seltzer and half a gallon of the juice (*laying down*). I strongly encourage you to get all of these items.

Even if you end up not using them, you will have them there just in case. Of course, if you are experienced in juice fasting, then you can simply follow whatever method works best for you. Okay, now it is time for you to stop reading and go to the supermarket. Please do it now or, if you cannot (*because it is 3:00 am!*) then do so over the next 24-hours at the very latest.

Chapter 13
Preparing to Juice

Let's get down to business! How did it go with the shopping? If this is your first time shopping strictly for fruits and vegetables, it may have been a little challenging. But it does get easier and, believe me, what you are doing here has the potential to literally alter the course of your life. <u>Remember</u>: the challenge you are now undergoing is part of the road you have resolved to travel to produce the weight loss and improved health you want. You may be going through some struggle **NOW**, but the benefits you will gain **LATER** will more than outweigh this temporary discomfort. With all the ingredients at hand, it is now time to prepare ourselves for the juicing process.

The Juicer

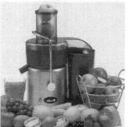

If you are already experienced using a juicer, then proceed with the preparation instructions below. If not, then let me take a moment to acquaint you. Most juicers have a primary pouring spout that releases the juice extracted from the fruits and vegetables.

Some more expensive models capture the juice in their own compartment for later pouring. If you have the former, then you will need an 8-to-12-ounce glass to place underneath the spout to capture the liquid as it comes out.

Moreover, you will need the one-gallon jug to store and refrigerate the juice. We will also need the aluminum foil to wrap the jug and protect the juice from the light in the refrigerator which can prematurely spoil the precious liquid. I know that sounds silly since the fridge is usually closed and dark. But I actually have had juice spoil prematurely and it is very disheartening. So stick with me. I won't lead you wrong, I promise!

Another section of the juicer that I want you to notice is the *"waste"* compartment where the pulp from the fruits and vegetables is discharged. Do you see it? I recommend that, for easier cleaning and disposal, you place a plastic bag (*I use small supermarket bags*) inside this partition as one would put a bag inside a trash can. That way all you have to do when you're done is remove the bag, close it and discard the leftovers. **Vegetable and fruit pulp spoils rapidly and can create a foul odor.** <u>Note</u>: There is really nothing *"wasteful"* about pulp, however. It has huge amounts of fiber and some of it is even tasty. We are actually going to scoop some of the pulp and mix it with the juice to help with bowel movements and detoxification! If you are unsure about where the pulp compartment is located in your juicer, refer to the instructions manual of the model that you purchased. Assembly is finalized by snapping in place the top cover over the liquefying blades. This cover normally includes the vertical feed opening where the produce is inserted. Once the top snaps into place, you will then be left with a plastic or wooden *"pusher tool"* that is used **to press the fruit and/or vegetable down the feed and into the grinder for liquefaction**.

Take a moment and review the parts I have just mentioned. Get acquainted with your juicer. By all means, make sure to read **ALL** of the instructions that came with your particular hardware. If you just purchased it, make sure to wash each part thoroughly with soap and water <u>prior</u> to assembly. This is important. I recall once juicer I purchased years ago, upon close inspection, had rotten chunks of fruit and vegetable on the cover and blades. Apparently it had been used, returned and nobody bothered to clean it. It was just dropped back in the aisles. Gross! Clean, clean, clean that juicer very thoroughly before you do anything else.

Once the juicer is ready and you have become familiar with how it works, then it is time to set it in place. Find the place in your kitchen counter where you intend to put the juicer. Find the largest possible area near an electric outlet. Now place a large towel <u>(or two)</u> to cover that entire area, placing the juicer on top of the towels. Using those towels will help a lot to minimize the mess. In addition, some of the darker-colored fruits may stain the counter. Make sure that the towel(s) cover the entire counter area where you will be juicing.

Prepping The Produce

Take the fruits and vegetables out of the refrigerator and place them on the kitchen counter. For now, leave them in the containers (or bags) in which you purchased them. Do this as close to the sink as possible. Take out the two bowls I mentioned earlier and set them aside. Also take out the cutting board and sharp knife for dicing and peeling. As I said earlier, you don't want to peel and cut the produce on the bare kitchen counter as you may scratch it. If you have a fruit/vegetable peeler, then use that. Now we are ready to start prepping the produce for juicing. Let's take them one by one:

Celery: Rip four sticks of celery from the stalk and wash them thoroughly with warm water. Celery stalks often contain traces of dirt in them. Once they are clean, place them in one of the bowls.

Tomatoes – Take two out, wash them and cut them in half. Place the four halves in the bowl.

Broccoli – Cut off a medium-sized chunk from the head including the stem. Rinse it in water and place it in the bowl.

Watercress – Rinse a medium hand full and set it on the bowl.

Carrots – Take three out of the bag. Shred the top layer of skin from each carrot by holding it diagonally in the sink and running the knife vertically from top to bottom as a scraper. You can also use a potato peeler. Once the carrots have been scraped, wash them thoroughly in warm water and place them in the bowl.

Pumpkin – Cut off a medium-sized piece of pumpkin from the chunk you purchased and use the knife to clean out the seeds and filling in the middle. Peel the outer skin with the knife or peeler and then place it in the bowl. (I still use a knife for peeling but I recognize that a peeler is probably easier). I guess I'm just set on my ways!

Apples – Take three out of the bag, wash them very thoroughly and cut them in half. Remove the seeds from the middle and place them in the bowl. Do not peel away the skin from the apples as it will create some good pulp!.

Blueberries & Strawberries – Wash a handful of blueberries and four strawberries and place them in the bowl whole. You don't have to cut the strawberries, but make sure to remove the green leaves on top.

Oranges – Take two oranges, wash, peel and cut them in half. Place the four halves in the bowl.

Lemons – Take out one lemon and cut it in half. We are not going to put the lemon in the juicer. Instead, we will squeeze the juice manually into the jar once all the other fruits and vegetables have been juiced.

The reason for this is that juicing the lemon, I have found, often makes the final juice way too acidic which can cause stomachaches. It is better to use lemons like salt and just season it to taste AFTER the juice is done.

Bananas – Take one-and-a-half bananas, peel them and place them in a separate cup or bowl. Bananas cannot be juiced. When the time comes, pour a cup of water in the blender along with the bananas and blend away until it liquefies. Then add the banana juice extract directly into the jug or jar with the final juice preparation. This will be the last step.

Once you are done with the peeling and cutting, you will have an amazing site in front of you: **a bowl overflowing with beautiful fruits and vegetables ready to enter and cleanse your body!** Look at the bowl for a minute and ponder at the wonderful benefit that you are about to receive.

Let the site fill you with the vision of health and weight loss that you have for your life. I realize that getting to this point required some work. You may have never done anything like this before.

You might even have had to overcome apathy, depression and/or discouragement (*among others*) to get up and actually take the action. My first time juicing was not a very joyous occasion. It took a **LOT** of push to make myself do it because I was so disgusted with my weight and health. Maybe you have been ill.

Maybe you have tried many different paths and nothing has worked. Yet <u>you are here</u>. You have shown willingness. Congratulations! Keep it up! I feel proud and honored to have you with me!

The Pusher or 'Guiding' Tool

We are now ready to juice the fruits and vegetables. There really is no order or science as to how you should juice. I juice fruits and vegetables in random order as I grab them from the bowl. The best way to start is with celery which is by far the vegetable with the most juice. From there you can simply continue with whatever fruit or vegetable is in front of you.

About the *"pusher or guiding tool."* As I mentioned earlier, most juicers come with a plastic or wooden tool that is used to guide the fruits and or vegetables into the feeder. **It is very important that you know how to use it properly or you will reduce the yield of juice**. We do not want to waste any of this precious juice! **<u>DO NOT</u>** push down on the tool! Once you insert a piece of produce into the feeder, allow it to go down at its own pace. Simply use the tool to "guide" the produce down to the grinder. **DO NOT FORCE IT!** The **MORE TIME** each piece of produce takes to make it down the feeder and into the blades, the **MORE JUICE** you will get. Use the pushing tool as a guide and do not force it! Always Remember: **MORE TIME = MORE JUICE.** In some cases, as with cauliflower or broccoli stems, you may need to push

"<u>LIGHTLY</u>" to ease the stress on the juicer blades. The same can sometimes happen with oranges, pumpkin and carrots. But, for the most part, you should <u>minimize the pressure</u> you exert on this tool. Allow the fruit or vegetable to make it through the feed on its own as much as possible. Use the guiding tool to follow the produce down the feed, but <u>push down on it only when necessary</u>.

Chapter 14
The Juicing Process

So, when you are ready:

Place the 8-to-10-ounce glass under the juicer spout to collect the liquid. Be sure to place some napkins or paper towels underneath the glass to absorb any spillage. Turn on the juicer and let it warm up for twenty seconds.

Then, take the first piece of celery and put it into the feeder. It will start grinding and bouncing around, getting smaller and smaller until it disappears into the blades. Observe the light green juice coming out of the spout and into the glass.

Now let's try a chunk of apple. Insert it into the feeder and follow it with the guiding tool into the blades. You will not get as much juice as you did with the celery, but watch it come out. Get used to the different color liquid that goes with each fruit and vegetable.

Life, Weight Loss & Healing

The juice you are seeing come out are fruits and vegetables in their purest form! It is life, weight loss, healing ... optimum health, mental clarity, detoxification, energy ... it is, in essence, <u>your own personal fountain of youth</u>. Let these thoughts enter your mind as you continue the juicing process.

At this point simply move on to the next fruit or vegetable in the bowl and repeat the process. As I said, carrots, pumpkin, oranges and broccoli may need a little push down. For leafy produce like watercress, sprinkle little bunches into the feeder. You will see the little spurts of dark green juice coming out of the spout and into the glass. Whenever you see that the glass is getting full, turn off the juicer and pour the liquid into the one-gallon jug you purchased.

But, **MAKE SURE** that you have an empty glass to place under the spout immediately as some juice will continue to ooze out **even after the juicer is turned off**. We want to capture that also! Then turn the juicer back on and continue the process. For blueberries, simply pour a handful into the feeder. **Strawberries can be fed whole.** Continue emptying the contents of the 8-ounce glass into the jug, always turning off the juicer and putting the *"backup"* glass under the spout to capture any dripping.

Pay close attention and do not allow any of the juice to spill! Inevitably there will always be some spillage, but it should be minor. **DO NOT** juice while you are *"multitasking"* - talking on the phone, watching television, or when otherwise being interrupted or distracted. This is a precious and *"sacred"* time for you and it should be treated as such! Focus on what you are doing! Once you have completely juiced all of the produce into the bowl, turn off the juicer and observe the *"fruits"* of your labor.

If you used a half-gallon jug, it should be almost full, or halfway if you utilized a gallon container. I never get tired of just looking at the multi-colored liquid as it sits in the container. Now that is pure power!

Adding the Pulp

Let the juice breathe uncovered for a few minutes. Unsnap the top of the juicer and direct your attention to the *"waste"* or pulp compartment. You will see the *"pasty"* leftovers of the fruits and vegetables. **That is far from garbage**. It is pure fiber which is great for the belly! Scoop two tablespoons of pulp and dump them into the juice. **You may want to eat a few spoonfuls. I love it.** Now, remove the plastic bag from the pulp compartment and zip it closed. I recommend that you **DO NOT** let this bag sit with your kitchen trash. Take it outside until garbage day. Some persons who enjoy gardening actually use it as fertilizer. I am not a gardener and have never tried this. But I have heard it works very well. Next, grab the lemons you cut earlier and squeeze their juice into the jug or jar. I do it manually, but if you have an extractor, by all means use it.

Banana Juice

Moving along, pour a cup of water into the blender along with the bananas and blend away! You should add plenty of water - one full glass of water for each banana. Banana juice tends to be a bit slimy, so we need it to be as liquid as possible so that it mixes well with the rest of the juice.

Thirty seconds in the blender is more than enough. Once finished, pour the banana juice into the jug with the rest of the juice. With a large wooden spoon or other utensil, stir the contents of the jug for about 15 seconds. **YOU ARE DONE**! Grandma would be proud!

Cleaning the Juicer

Now it is time for what probably is the least enjoyable part of the process: <u>cleaning the juicer</u>. Leave the juice uncovered and turn your attention to disassembling the juicer and placing its parts in the sink. Most juicers come with a small brush for cleaning. Make sure to unplug the juicer before you start disassembling it! You can probably rinse most of it off, but it is VERY IMPORTANT that you spend as much time as needed **brushing the blades and removing every last trace of pulp**. When you are done, the blades should look as though they were never used! Do not cut corners. Dirty blades lose their sharpness quicker, and **even small traces of pulp can rot and contaminate any juices you prepare in the future.** Wipe down the main juicer, ensuring that all traces of juice have been cleaned. When you are satisfied the cleaning has been thorough, set the juicer parts aside to dry.

Finish the cleaning process by removing the towel from the kitchen counter, wiping off any spillage and grinding any fruit or vegetable skin (*that you peeled earlier*) in your garbage disposal. Follow this system <u>every time</u> you juice.

It is best to clean right away while you are giving the juice time to breathe. That way, when the time comes to drink, you can do so in peace without having to worry about doing any cleaning.

Chapter 15
Handling & Tasting the Juice

During the cleanup process, you set the juice aside to breathe. Now, screw the lid tightly on the jug. Make sure that it is tight and that no juice will spill. Then turn it upside down and shake it vigorously for about 30 seconds. It is amazing to see the pulp mix with the rest of the juice, leaving a layer of foam at the top. At this point, if the jug is not completely full, you can cap it with more water and the vegetable juice you purchased. But don't add too much vegetable juice. One glass of water and one glass of vegetable juice should be more than enough to fill the gallon jug nearly to the top. If not, that is fine. You've done a great job.

Now to the best part of all ... drinking the juice! Fill a glass with the juice and have a taste! Drink it slowly, visualizing the powerful healing nutrients entering your bloodstream and digestive system – cleaning and wiping out toxins in their path! Most people love the taste of the juice. If you do not, then don't worry about it. It will grow on you. The next time you juice, you can start to add a bit more or less of certain produce. Eventually, you will find the taste that works best for you. But this is not about focusing on the taste. Watercress tends to be bitter, especially if you have never had it before. Or some other unusual taste may stand out. Give it time and focus on the benefits that you're gaining in weight loss and health.

If you have spent years eating a lot of unhealthy junk, then this is truly a gourmet feast that your body is **VERY** thankful to receive.

Now, screw the lid tightly on the jug again. Take out the aluminum foil and cover the entire jug as if you were wrapping a present. What better gift to your life than this, right? Once sealed, place the jug in the refrigerator. It is best to place it in a spacious location where the jug doesn't have to be constantly moved to access other items in the refrigerator. We want the juice to be protected and secure at all times.

If there are young children at home, I suggest that you instruct them not to handle the jug on their own as they may drop it or otherwise spill it. But, by all means, give them a taste! If you can get them used to drinking pure fruits and veggies when they're still young, you will be giving them one of the best gifts that they could receive.

Chapter 16
Choose a Start Date

Well, we have covered a lot of ground, looked at the power of fruits and vegetables, done the shopping, prepared the juice and now are ready to jump into the actual process of fasting. The juice that you prepared needs to be consumed in no longer than three days. So it is important at this point for you to begin the fast as quickly as possible - no later than 24 hours from now. This is very exciting. I almost feel as though I am right there with you in person... sharing a moment that - *without a doubt* - is sure to have a great impact on your life. Right now, we must press on with the task at hand. There is much reward in this, but there is also a lot of challenge. Therefore, the most important step you can take now is to: **CHOOSE A START DATE**.

Mark your calendar and propose to yourself that **THAT** will be the day when you begin your 30-day fast. I like to start on Sundays because it gives me a straight week-to-week structure. However, your schedule may be different. As a rule, it is preferable to start the fast during your 'weekend,' or whichever time you have weekly of least activity. That way you can get plenty of rest in the initial days of the fast before you have to resume any type of work schedule or other. **IF**, you are able to take the entire month off to focus strictly on fasting, then THAT would be the best case scenario.

If you work, maybe you have enough time off available to at least take one or two weeks off. Anything would be fine. Should the opportunity to take time off be available to you, I encourage you to seize it. If not, then that is fine. I have done plenty of long-term fasts while maintaining an active (*and very demanding*) schedule. It is doable. In some cases, it is even better **because you will be busy and time will go by faster**. So please don't put off this task if you do work a full-time job. If I did it, so can you. And you will have plenty of juice as nourishment, so you will not be totally abstaining from all food as one would during a total water fast. You might not have as much energy as you normally would, but you still will be able to make it through. **So: did you choose a start date? Excellent! You have taken yet another step towards the realization of your goals.**

Chapter 17
Pre-Fasting Steps

The 5 'D's

Let me share with you the five key steps (*which I call the Five D's*) that helped me to hang on, even when the symptoms and hunger were at their worst. Take your time and put these to practice thoroughly as I know that they will help you a lot. The point of these five steps is to give you the strongest foundation possible for your fast. So don't skip through these or take them lightly please!

DECIDE that you are through with the old way of things. Look at the goals that you have related to your health, weight and eating. Resolve in your heart-of-hearts that you **ARE** going to follow through - no matter what. Draw an imaginary line that ends your old way of eating and relating to food, health and wellness, and become totally willing in your inner self to take the action to change **PERMANENTLY** – one day at a time.

DEFINE the type of life that you want to have as a result of your new healthy lifestyle. Look at the new avenues, activities and relationships you want to engage in as you move forward. So, as of now, (*if you haven't done so already*) mark that calendar and decide when you intend to start the juice fast. If you have truly defined the type of life that you want for yourself, then moving forward with your goals is an absolute must.

And I'm not talking about tomorrow, next week or next month. I am talking about **RIGHT HERE AND RIGHT NOW!**.

DECLARE to your close friends and family that you are through with being overweight and toxic and that you will be implementing some changes during the next months to lose weight and get. Tell them that you will **<u>NO LONGER</u>** be indulging in junk food and that you do not wish for it to be offered. The purpose of this step is to give you some immediate accountability with persons that know you. It is not the same to sneak a pizza when nobody knows what you are doing! You do not, however, have to disclose your plans to everyone. Disclose it only to immediate family members, of course... people that you trust and you know will not judge or try to put banana peels in your path. You may not realize it, but there are people who may actually resent that you are taking action to get a hold of your life and health. Be aware and don't let them bring you down!

DESIGNATE a specific person that you trust and tell him or her specifically what you intend to do and why. Ask this person for support during the process and stay accountable to him or her on a regular basis. Visit **FitnessThroughFasting.com** and visit the forums where you can give and receive lots of support and motivation. There are tons of online forums dedicated to weight loss. Find one that you feel comfortable in and make it a point to get involved with the community. That alone will help you in more ways that you can imagine.

In short, this step is designed so that you can determine which person in your close circle would best be suited to support you in the coming nine-months.

DEVELOP a strong journal where you can put in writing the reasons why it is important **FOR YOU** to reach your weight loss goals. Some examples can be; *weight loss, better health, healing from specific illnesses, more energy and vitality, mental clarity, dropping clothing sizes to a particular size, participating in a certain sport, getting married, dating, wearing a bathing suit you always wanted to, having a flat stomach, getting into your high-school-days clothing etc...* These are personal reasons and are crucial because they mean something **TO YOU**... not to your spouse, children or family... but **TO YOU**! Yes, our loved ones are an immense source of motivation to get us going, but ultimately we have to do this **FOR OURSELVES.**

I cannot stress enough the importance of keeping a journal. In it, you can write the **dreams and goals that are closest to your he**art. You can write exactly what you want to get out of your weight loss efforts. **And those dreams and goals are the powerhouse of your spirit and min**d. Each time you find yourself weak and wanting to give in, you can pick up the journal and read what you have written. During those moments of weakness, **REMEMBER** the huge payoff in health and weight loss that you will receive. Learn that "a *life worth living is a life worth recording.*"

Chapter 18
Intermittent Fasting
Alternatives

I get into much more detail about intermittent fasting on <u>Volume 5</u> of this series titled **The Intermittent Fasting Weight Loss Formula**, so I encourage you to purchase and read that book as well when you have a chance. I also encourage you to check out <u>Volume 1</u> **The Permanent Weight Loss Diet**.' That book goes into great detail with dieting. It can help you lose more weight as well as help you to establish good eating habits. As guidance, however, here are some intermittent fasting choices that you can consider. Not everyone may be ready to fast nonstop for an entire 30 days. However, there are shorter fasts that you can start to practice right way so that you can build experience, strength and confidence. Let's take a look at what these options are:

Daily Intermittent Fasting: As in Catholic Lent Fasting and Muslim Ramadan, here you would fast from sunup to sundown - approximately 12 hours daily. The fast is broken each night with a light meal, preferably of lean fish or poultry, small portion of carbs (4oz baked or sweet potato) and steamed veggies. Your "eating window" remains open until dawn, but for most of that time you will be sleeping. Twelve hours to eat, twelve hours to fast... and so the cycle continues each day.

You can get up in the AM, have breakfast, and then fast for the next 12 hours. I love Daily (IF). It is great for beginners.

After acquiring some experience, many like to add hours as they are motivated. In the beginning, you may be adding minutes. That's OK. Minutes add up to hours and hours add up to days. Remember, progress not perfection. In other words, certain days you may feel great and want to fast for another few hours. That is fine. But try not to exceed 16 hours of fasting each day, so as to not interrupt the Daily (IF) cycle. Estimated Weekly weight loss: three to five pounds.

Every Other Day Intermittent Fasting: Another form of intermittent fasting is to go for an entire 24-hour cycle every other day. Example: You fast from 8am Monday morning to 8am Tuesday morning. Eat lightly on Tuesday in observance of the SLD. Wake up on Wednesday at 7:30am and have breakfast. Start the fast at 8am until the same time on Thursday... and so on. Estimated Weekly weight loss: two to four pounds.

Half Week Intermittent Fasting: Fast for 3.5 days of the week. Example: Fast from 8am Monday to 8pm Thursday. You can return to regular eating for the rest of the week. Fasting would resume the following Monday at 8am - repeating the same cycle. This system requires caution, however. Since one does not eat for 84-hour periods, it will be necessary to follow the breaking a fast instructions, listed towards the end of this book.

Estimated weekly weight loss: three to five pounds.
Seven Day Intermittent Fasting: Fast for an entire seven days, return to your regular diet for seven days, and then fast for another seven days. Similar to the Half Week method, you will need follow the breaking a fast instructions. Estimated weekly weight loss: Five to 20 pounds during initial 7-day fast and five to seven on subsequent ones.

Combination Intermittent Fasting: The ultimate way to practice intermittent fasting is to combine all of the above and complete 14 and 30-day cycles of intermittent fasts. Combination can also be doing 24-hour juice fasting once a week, three-day juice fasting weekly or bi-weekly... whatever is within your ability to do, THAT is more than enough to get started. As I said already, what matters is that you jump aboard and get going. By no means pressure yourself to do a long fast that you aren't mentally prepared to do. A lot of people that have fasted for 14 days and beyond first had to begin with shorter ones to build their stamina. So, if you are experienced and have done it before, then bon voyage - you're on your way. If, on the other hand, you are new to juice fasting, then do what you can and build from there. No matter what you are able to do, you come off a winner!

Chapter 19
Starting the Fast

Now the moment of truth has arrived. The time has come to take action and begin your journey. The juice is ready... let's get the ball rolling! I am going to assume at this point that you are prepared to start fasting <u>tomorrow</u>. So today is the last day of your *'pre-fasting'* life. From this point forward, you will be entering the land of miracles. The possibilities for your health and wellness are unlimited. You have worked hard and made it this far.

Spend some time today writing on your journal. Get used to writing about your thoughts and feelings. Set your schedule and make a firm commitment with yourself that you will hang on to the end **NO MATTER WHAT**. You have had plenty of time to prepare, so there should be no *'surprises'* that this point to sidetrack you. Rain or shine, you are going to make it **ALL THE WAY** and give yourself this amazing gift of life and health. <u>**NOTHING**</u> is more important than what you are doing here. The rest of your life begins now. Are you ready?

Let's move forward with the motivational messages, starting on **Day 0** which is <u>**TODAY**</u>, the day before the fast.

Chapter 20
Motivational Messages

The messages I have put together here will guide you day-by-day through the first 10 days of the fasting process. The best way to use them is to read each one at the start of each day, and then continue to re-read the message as the hours go by. Once you reach day 10, start again at day one... and so on until you complete the fast. I have handpicked these messages from my archives and they are the ones that readers have found most useful.

Use these messages and keep them close at all times. I am certain that they will help you a lot. There actually are a total of 11 messages, starting with the day **BEFORE** you start the fast. So, start with **Day 0** once you are ready to begin. You're on your way to losing a lot of weight very quickly and drastically improving your health and quality of life. Here we go:

Day 0 - Day Before the Fast

The fact that you are reading these words shows that you are committed to doing whatever it takes to improve your health and quality of life. Am I right? Are you prepared to put to practice what you have learned and see this all the way through? I believe that you are! *And for that I say*: Congratulations and welcome to your fast! If you have never fasted before, you are in for quite the ride. If you **HAVE** done long-term fasts before, then I am certain you will learn even more as we go from day to day.

These messages are designed to "*accompany*" you through this fast. I want you to feel that I am beside you every step of the way. **This is how it's going to work**: For the duration of your fast, open this book and read the next motivational message. There are a total of 10 messages, excluding this one that you are reading. When you reach the tenth message, start again with message one the next day. By then, *if you have decided to go longer than 11 days*, you will have gone through the toughest part of the fast. The messages will continue to reinforce the task at hand and take you to the end of the fast. I will mention what you may be going through, things to watch out for, and, I'll give you plenty of encouragement. Also, as mentioned in *'The 5 D's,'* be sure to spend as much time as possible writing in your journal. The thoughts, feelings and perspectives that you will receive as you move forward will prove invaluable in the future.

In writing, you could very well achieve a profound emotional breakthrough. I have journals from fasts I did three, five, ten years ago and - *let me tell you* - I **ALWAYS** get a lot when I revisit them.

For today: Have your last meal at around 8PM, drink two large glasses of water and go to bed. We will make it... just one moment, one day at a time. Get plenty of rest tonight. I will talk to you in the morning!

Day 1

We are off and running. The first day is one of adapting physically and mentally. You ate your final meal last night, so you already have been fasting for at least 12 hours. That means that the hunger will come very soon. Be ready! Before we go any further, please stop reading and go have two large glasses of water. Make it a point to drink at least half a gallon daily, one gallon would be even better! **Water is your ally** and will help soothe hunger and detox symptoms. Read the chapter below for more detail on the symptoms that you may experience while fasting.

You can drink your first 8-to-12-ounce glass of juice one hour after you wake up. When you are ready to drink, pour the juice from the jug and sit down to 'eat.' Don't just drink the juice nonchalantly. Make sure to breathe and take your time. Chew the pulp well and taste those nutrients that your body is taking in. You can have another glass of juice every **FOUR** hours, totaling no more than 64 ounces per day (*eight, 12-ounce portions*).

Spend time in your fasting journal and get used to writing your thoughts and feelings. **Nothing is too silly**. You may find yourself writing just a few words. You may find yourself writing a lot. Maybe profanity is all that will come out. So be it. Journal it. You can start to clear your thoughts right away; begin to focus more on what you are thinking and feeling... "*the inner world*". Writing will help you.

If you have religious or spiritual beliefs, take some time (*after you drink the morning juice*) and say a prayer... ask for strength and guidance.

Remind yourself why you are fasting, and why you are choosing to complete this process. This is **NOT** a game or some half-measured step. You have specific and strong reasons for doing this, and it has to do with **transforming your life for the better**, right? You want to lose weight, get healthy and rejuvenate! Make sure to speak to your **DECLARE** and **DESIGNATE** support buddy at some point during the day. I have found that afternoons are best because that is the time when hunger and symptoms hit me the most. This entire fast will go by faster and smoother is you have someone who supports and is there for you (*apart from me!*). Please follow this suggestion. You won't regret it.

If you leave the house daily *(to work, errands, etc)*, please make sure you pack your cooler with plenty of ice, a few bottles of drinking water, two bottles of seltzer (*sparkling water, club soda*). If you will be gone for less than four hours, take no less than 16 ounces of juice with you in case you are detained for whatever reason. The juice is your lifeline and you must have it close at all times. If you intend to be away all day, then fill the half-gallon jug with 32 ounces of juice, enough to cover you a full eight hours. Always make sure to close the lid tightly. Place it into the cooler. It may not fit in the cooler standing up. In such a case, place it in the cooler horizontally with the rest of your supplies.

You should always have these items with you when you leave the house. That is why I told you that the ice cooler comes in very handy. If you feel silly carrying the cooler around, don't worry about it. Do it anyways.

When away, also **take with you at least four bags of green tea**. When hunger strikes, have **two large glasses of water**. Crack open a bottle of seltzer. Around noon have a cup of green tea. Try to stay busy, but take it easy physically. Brace yourself; the hunger pains will come and often be strong. Drink more water, seltzer... green tea as well as your glass of juice every four hours. In the afternoon, you also may start to feel detox symptoms; weakness, dizziness, nausea, headaches, irritability, white coat on tongue, metallic taste in mouth. Drink more water, seltzer... green tea. **Move slowly, take a nap if you can**.

On average, hunger and symptoms will diminish (and even vanish) after around 14 days of juice fasting. All in all, after two weeks you should be feeling a lot better. So keep that target in mind as you move forward. Stick to the plan; I'll be here with you. Don't just read this message <u>ONCE</u> and then move on. Use it! Read it, read it, read it! :-)

There is no more time to waste. This is YOUR time. This is the time of your change and transformation. And it has already begun... Remember, the "discomfort is a sign that you are getting better". It doesn't feel good, but the health and weight loss benefits that will result make this "small sacrifice" worth its weight in gold! In the evening, watch TV, read a book, write some closing thoughts on your journal.

Right now, say to yourself: *"Just for today, no matter what, no matter what, no matter what, I am NOT going to eat. I am going to stick to my fast and I am going to finish what I started. I thank the God of my understanding for giving me the strength and resolve I need to make it. I am grateful that fasting will make me healthier, leaner and more vibrant so I can be more effective and useful to my loved ones and others."*

Day 2

Welcome to **DAY TWO** of your 30-day fast. I hope you got plenty of sleep. I find that, when I fast, I sleep very deeply and wake up refreshed. Some people, however, go through periods of insomnia, restlessness and even nightmares. This is due to the **release of toxins into the bloodstream and will pass**. If you find yourself struggling to sleep, I recommend that you drink some soothing Chamomile tea at night before you retire. You can find it at most supermarkets, or you can order it at amazon.com. If you still cannot sleep, take a tryptophan or valerian root tablet.

As you did yesterday, drink two large glasses of water as soon as you wake up. Drinking plenty of water during the day will help to expedite the *"flush-out"* of the toxins from your body. Usually, hunger will be minimal in the mornings when you first wake up. Enjoy it. Over the following hours you will start to notice the pangs start to increase - so **be very careful today**. Remain vigilant. It is during this early phase that most tend to give up. As usual, drink your first glass of juice one hour after you wake up. Every four hours you are due an eight-to-12-ounce glass of juice. Yes, you are getting to know the drill, right? Apart from the physical symptoms, also pay close attention to your mind and emotions. Learn to identify and reject all thoughts, arguments, rationalizations and justifications the mind may give you to give up.

Resistance, resistance, resistance is key at this phase! None of the discomfort should come as a big shock to you.

We knew it would be a challenge. But you can make it through. I know that you can. **DAY TWO** is nearly-always a day of battle. But you know what you have to do. Write in your journal, review past lessons, drink plenty of water, pray, meditate... whatever it takes to keep you busy and moving forward.

Visit the various forums at **FitnessThroughFasting.co**m and find as many people as you can to motivate and comfort. It never ceases to amaze me just how powerful this simple practice is. You can be almost collapsing from hunger and/or detox symptoms, yet a few minutes writing to help someone else and you'll be strengthened and refreshed. The more time you spend *"giving"* strength, the more you will receive! Not to mention that you will find plenty of people there to support and comfort you as well. Those forums are immensely helpful. Go there daily and get involved. You may even find me there! :-)

Every time, every moment that hunger and detox symptoms disturb you, remember this: **YOU ARE NOT GOING THROUGH THE DISCOMFORT IN VAIN!** You have a plan and you have the courage. You are taking control of your life and squashing anything that stands in your way. **You are adding quality years to your life and bravely going through the road less-traveled.**

Every symptom **MUST** yield to your resolve. This, without a doubt, is one of the most important moments in your life. Do you see it! Can you internalize the **HUGE** magnitude of what you are doing? Try to take it easy if you are able. Stay busy but <u>do not</u> put yourself through unnecessary exertion. You may start to experience some mood *swings now; irritability, sadness, hopelessness, anger, rage... these are all symptoms that you are getting better.* The toxins are being wiped out and your mind and emotions are also undergoing a process of purging and healing.

Thank the God of your understanding and ask for strength to make it through. This is **NOT** just about losing weight and external physical health. You also have put yourself in a position to undergo profound emotional healing and spiritual growth. The benefits are huge! And, remember, **the symptoms will pass. The hurricane will weaken. You will reach the shore a stronger and more vibrant person.**

Say to yourself: *"Just for today, I will keep in mind that I am undergoing a physical, mental and spiritual cleansing and will not react when I feel bad. I will let the symptoms and feelings pass and keep my eyes <u>ONLY</u> on reaching my goals. I will ask the God of my understanding for help and be empowered by my choice to live a better life".*

Day 3

DAY THREE! Seventy-two hours... you are entering deeper and deeper waters. How have you been feeling? Have you been drinking plenty of water? Have you been writing in your journal? Did you call your **DESIGNATE** friend? If you have, then good for you! That shows commitment, courage and willingness. You will be greatly rewarded mentally, physically and, yes, spiritually.

Nothing kills our progress more than procrastination and closed-mindedness. So give yourself completely to this fast. I cannot overestimate the power that it will unleash in your life. Today can either be the toughest day of the fast, or it can be the day when one begins to feel better. It all depends on how your body reacts. But you are gaining ground. The digestive system is slowing down considerably and the body is starting to feed more and more on stored fat.

Ketosis is almost complete (*the process where the body shifts from feeding on food intake, to feeding mostly on stored fat*). Drink your customary two large glasses of water upon awakening, the eight-to-12-ounce glass of juice one hour later, and every four hours afterward.

Make sure that you have enough seltzer and decaffeinated green tea to carry you through the day. Those are your allies and we do not want to run short.

<u>About Green Tea</u>: Drinking pure oolong tea or green tea extract - *a more concentrated form of oolong tea* - will give you energy and calm physical discomfort. The green tea leaf has large quantities of phytochemical polyphenols called flavonols, known as <u>catchetins</u>. According to a recent green tea study by the Linus Pauling Institute at Oregon State University, green tea fosters weight loss because **the body starts using greater amounts of energy after it is consumed.**

This is a direct result of the catchetins' intrinsic fat oxidation and body heating properties. In short, green tea can help a lot. Have some baggies on you wherever you go so that you can offset that annoying afternoon sinking spell. But please make sure to only get decaf green tea if at all possible.

The juice may also be running low. At some point today, go through the juicing process again and make a fresh supply. You have my detailed instructions, so make sure to follow them. **Do not mix the old juice with the new**. Pour the juice that is left from three days ago into the half-gallon jug. Wash the gallon jug thoroughly. Fill it with hot water, close the lid and shake it vigorously to disinfect and make sure that all pieces of pulp are loosened. Pay close attention to the lid as a lot of residue tends to accumulate there. If you need to go to the store for more supplies, <u>take a friend with you</u>. Or maybe somebody else can go for you.

Stay away from food and eating establishments as much as possible.

This is a crucial time in the fast. The worst of the toxins are being eliminated; that is what causes the symptoms and the hunger pangs. You **KNOW** why you are doing this. You are determined to make it to the other side. You are tired of talking about it and wishing and sighing... *"you are prepared to take the action and to stay the course until you produce the results that you want"*. Am I right? Your body is busy cleansing and healing. **All you have to do is stay put and give it the time it needs to complete the process**. The weight loss accelerates today. The body is shifting to *"full fat-burning mode"* and a lot of toxins are being eliminated, along with the normal water weight loss. The toxins that have been hiding in stored fat are being exposed and wiped out.

You, your body *and the God of your understanding* are working together to vanquish these enemies and achieve ultimate health and breakthrough. And I am here cheering you on; filling **your mind with powerful thoughts and motivation! Say to yourself**: *"Just for today, I am going to surrender to the process and give my body the time that it needs to heal and cleanse. I thank the God of my understanding that I have been given the knowledge and strength I need to make it through these 24 hours. I am at peace and in full expectation of greater and greater blessings."*

Day 4

Hello dear friend, and welcome to day 4! It is very possible that today the hunger and detox symptoms will begin to subside. **OR**, as is the case with me, you may be in the middle of the storm and struggling to hang on. But you have the willingness to work through this challenge. I encourage you to spend as much time as possible in your journal.

We are not out of the woods yet and need to use everything at our disposal to make it from day to day. Good news: Your body will reach full Ketosis today. For many people, the hunger and detox symptoms are starting to subside. How are you feeling? Waking up with little or no hunger is one of the most rewarding times. Have you experienced that? If you have **NOT** felt any improvement and are struggling, just hang on! **It will pass, it will pass, it will pass! Did I mention also that it will pass?**

Just hang on, put on your armor and continue offering full **RESISTANCE**. Enough is enough right? You are **NOT** going to continue to give up years of your life without achieving the optimum health that you deserve. Get tough... get angry! What is going through your mind today? Are you spending time in your fasting journal? You are now in the midst of the full power of fasting. You are going deeper and deeper into the land of miracles.

Your spirit is more awake than ever ... whatever your spiritual belief, **NOW** is an amazingly-powerful moment to have communion with the *God of your understanding.* Spending more time in your accustomed prayers and/or meditation is highly encouraged.

Optimize water intake today. Make it a point to drink a **FULL** gallon of water daily for the remainder of the fast. You may already be drinking that much. If so, then keep doing it. If not, then today I want you to push yourself and force some more water down. Let's increase the flushing power flowing through your organs. Let's continue to support the body's fat-burning mission.

Wherever you go, don't forget to carry your cooler with water and seltzer. **Don't forget to take plenty of green tea to help you with energy.** Did you prepare the new batch of juice yesterday? How did it go? Remember, two glasses of water when you get up, your first eight-to-twelve-ounce glass of juice one hour later and every four hours thereafter. Do not drink more than 64 ounces of juice per day.

Be careful when getting up and moving. The weakness at this point of the fast may be very noticeable. You will probably feel **dizzy and may have difficulty getting around.** Rest is the best alternative. If you must move, do so slowly and do **NOT** make any sudden jerky movements. **Mental confusion and fogginess is also norma**l. The cleansing is deep ... do not become discouraged.

Here are the detox symptoms that you may experience in the first two weeks of the fast:

Headaches – This one is especially marked for coffee drinkers, but is also the case for persons who consume large amounts of sugar and alcohol. This symptom can really take a person out of commission. A lot of my colleagues call me a heretic for saying this, but if you need to take a couple of ibuprofen tablets to ease the pain, then so be it. Usually two tablets will do the trick. But don't take more than four daily. You may need to go through a little pain and discomfort. The good news is that headaches rarely last more than 72 hours, if that.

Dizziness – The body is not used to being deprived of eating whatever it wants and will go through dizzy spells, particularly during the first 11 days. The best solution for dizziness is to move slowly and get as much rest as your daily schedule allows.

Difficulty Performing Basic Tasks – Since you aren't consuming solid food, it will take some time for the body to adjust. You will more than likely feel very weak and may have trouble getting around - particularly during the first 10-14 days. If you slow down and work on focusing on the individual tasks you are performing, this symptom can be overcome. It is important for you to realize that your body is going through a transition. You must move slowly and not try to push yourself too hard. You may not be able to function at the same capacity as you are accustomed. Fine.

Slow down and give the body time to work on your behalf.

Weakness means that you need to be extra careful when walking around, and especially when getting up from a sitting position. Avoid harsh and/or abrupt movements. Move slowly, watch your step closely and always have something that you can hang on to if you suddenly feel like you are fainting. This is good advice. One time I totally hit the deck because I got up to quickly from a chair. I missed the corner of the wall by centimeters, but still hit myself quite hard on the floor. This is about improving our health, not about getting hurt. Please be careful. I mean it. Be careful.

Pulsating Hunger Pains that disappear and then re-emerge throughout the day. For some persons, hunger is monstrous in the morning. But for the vast majority, the hunger troll shows up mostly at night. More about night cravings below. In short, hunger will always be a part of our lives, and it is our task to master it rather than allow it to enslave us as it **CAN AND WILL** if we let it.

In my case, hunger was very strong in the first week to 10 days of juice fasting, and then I found myself getting used to always being 'a little' hungry. After a while, I loved it because I began to feel more alert, more energetic, optimistic... I slept better. I actually **SLEPT THROUGH THE NIGHT** and woke up feeling terrific. Before the juice fast, I constantly woke up at night to urinate, or like a raving lunatic wanting to raid the fridge.

After a while, I would go to sleep at 11PM, close my eyes and, when I opened them, it was 6AM! For me, this was nothing less than a total miracle. And I felt great... refreshed and ready to go! All of that just from getting used to eating less and being a little hungry. Much better than getting stuffed like a boar as I used to.

Bad Breath, Metallic Taste in Mouth, White Sticky Film on Tongue – These are all good indications that your body is eliminating toxicity. Most of these symptoms pass after 14 days (*on average*). **Bad Breath**, I suggest that you get sugarless mints and keep them handy until the process ends. **Metallic Taste In the Mouth** usually means that there are excessive (*and toxic*) heavy metals accumulated in your system. I recall during my first juice fast tasting constant sulfur and 'steel' in my mouth for like one week. **White Sticky Film on the Tongue** is completely repulsive but necessary. It's just another way for your body to get rid of all of the crap in your body that has kept you addicted to junk and overweight. For these symptoms, the best thing you can do is to keep drinking a lot of water. Make sure to brush your teeth regularly. Keep a travel toothbrush with you if you spend a lot of time out. Mouthwash is also helpful.

Diarrhea or Constipation – All of the fecal matter adhered to your colon will either start gushing out in diarrhea or incite short-term constipation. I know that this is disgusting, but it happens.

If you have eaten poorly for a long time, or have simply abused sugar or fat, your body may respond to the juice fast by expelling toxins in this fashion.

If Diarrhea Strikes, simply continue to follow the juice fast as outlined. Should it become severe, see your pharmacist and ask him or her for an over-the-counter recommendation. Continue with the juice fast. Fasting is a shock to the body, but it will finally get the message and react favorably to what you are doing. If you have diarrhea, make sure to keep yourself hydrated. Make it a point to drink at least one gallon of water daily. Stay close to a bathroom at all times. If you go out, make sure that you are always aware where the nearest restroom is. Seriously, you want to get to the toilet promptly anytime you need to.

If Constipation is The Case, visit your local pharmacy and ask your pharmacist about a stool softener. I personally use a herbal laxative called **Herbs & Prunes**. It works like a charm every time and is not harsh on my stomach. Take one tablet to start. Do not exceed four tablets in one day. But do this only if you fail to eliminate anything for at least three days. Give your body enough time to do it on its own.

Irritability / Mood Swings – If you have ever seen The Flintstones, you may remember Fred walking around growling on the episode where he is placed on a diet. Sooooo, be prepared to be a little *"short-fused"* during this time of heavy-duty preparation. Be aware that you will not be as patient as you normally would be.

Tell your loved ones not to take it personally if - initially - you are less social that what they are accustomed. **This is normal and will pass**.

Facial Puffiness & Feeling Bloated – This symptom is much more marked for persons who consume large amounts of salt and/or sugar. I personally was bloated to the max like the **Stay Puft Marshmallow man**. So being puffy was nothing new. I looked like somebody had stuck huge balloons on my cheeks. It was hideous. Juice fasting took care of that and my face today is that of a normal human being rather than a cartoon character.

That is a lot of symptoms, but rarely does **ONE** person experience them all. And remember, they will subside and mostly pass after approximately 14 days. Still, we discussed in the first chapters, the symptoms indicate that your body is cleansing, getting healthier and stronger. Continue to surrender to the process and stay put. Let the body do what it does best. Your body knows how to take care of you. Your body and digestive system thank you for this break. Your body is loyal and noble ... it is **unleashing amazing weight loss and healing power even as we speak**. All you have to do is hang on and let the process run its course.

Say to yourself: *"Just for today, I am going to stay on my fast no matter what my mind and body tell me. Today I am going to keep in mind constantly just how important this is to me and how many wonderful benefits I am gaining by staying the path.*

I thank the God of my understanding for giving me the strength and courage that I need. I trust the amazing task my body is doing on my behalf".

Day 5

WOW, DAY FIVE! You are amazing. How is it going? Each passing moment brings you closer to your ultimate goal. Did you speak to your **DESIGNATE** buddy and visit any forums? This is a priority. If you haven't done it, then please make sure to do so starting today. None of us are supermen. We need each other, and that is what the forums are all about. **Please follow my instructions**. Remember that <u>I have gone through this road before</u>. So whatever I ask you to do, it isn't 'just because.' I am asking you to do it because I have walked the path and know that it works.

Did you drink an entire gallon of water yesterday as I asked you? Make sure to do that, even if you do not feel thirsty or your body does not want it. Water intake is a crucial part of the cleansing process and it also helps expedite the passing of detox symptoms. Day **FIVE** can often be a day of much weakness, dizziness and medium-to-strong hunger pains. Although, in many cases hunger and symptoms have diminished by now.

How is it going with you? What would you say is causing the most discomfort; detox? Hunger? Both? Make sure to write all of this information down in your fasting journal. That will give you excellent insight of how your body reacts when fasting. When you do another long-term fast in the future, you will know what to expect. Such information is invaluable. So write, write, write! Today I want you to spend time writing in the journal.

Just put pen to paper and start to write what is in your heart and mind. You are amidst a dynamic program of change. NOW is an amazing time. We are reflecting on the past, present and future. What you are going through is but **a tiny micro in comparison to the large scheme of things and your life as a whole**. In fact, the discomfort that you may be feeling has the potential to "*make the remaining years of your life drastically-more vibrant and effective*". Keep your eyes on **THAT** prize. It is more than a prize... **it is a treasure**!

Again, you are **NOT** walking through the discomfort of fasting because you like it. NO! You are going through the wilderness because, just slightly ahead, there is "*a promised land of weight loss and improved health that will take you to unprecedented levels of physical, mental and spiritual freedom*". I want you to **SEE** that promised land.

Say to yourself: "*Just for today, I will continue with the fast with eyes firmly-fixed on my health-improvement goals. I will spend time in my journal taking stock of my life. I will ask the God of my understanding to show me what I need to see and grant me the spirit of revelation. I believe that I am being healed physically, mentally and spiritually and am grateful for the beautiful gifts I am receiving through fasting*".

Day 6

We are now at **DAY SIX**! Regardless of how you may be feeling today, six days of fasting is an amazing accomplishment. **By now you have walked through the very worst of the fast and have confronted your human weaknesses in ways you may have never done before**. You will definitely walk away a much stronger and sharper person as a result of what you are doing.

At around day **FIVE**, roughly 80% of the "*surface*" toxins in the bloodstream and digestive system have been eliminated. So today you may be feeling "*a little*" better. But there is still another round of symptoms coming up. I want you to be ready. Around **DAY SIX**, the body starts to dig into the "*deep*" toxins that "*hide*" inside muscles and stored fat. These are the worst of the worst and, consequently, cause the harshest of the hunger pangs and detox symptoms.

This phase lasts until day 10 to day 14, at which point symptoms and hunger will diminish. Remember, some people may experience hunger and symptoms for <u>as long as 21 days</u> - depending on overall health and level of toxicity. If this is the case with you, **DO NOT BE DISCOURAGED**! It will pass, it will pass, it will pass! Oh, and I forgot to tell you: it will pass! Hang in there... <u>you are well on your way</u>. You've come way too far to give up now!
If you weigh yourself today, **it is probable that you may have lost as in excess of 10 pounds**.

How much weight have you lost? Log it in the fasting journal. **The fastest daily average of weight loss happens over the initial 7 days of fasting.** However, the fat burning machine continues. Even now, as you read this, your body is eating away stored fat and making you leaner and healthier!

Weakness and dizziness usually linger. Sometimes these symptoms are such that one can hardly move. That is normal. Again, rest is the best way to handle it. If you can spend most of your time relaxing, reading, writing and maybe watching a few good movies; that would be best. Please **DO NOT** make any plans that require too much activity. Once more, I remind you to drink at least **ONE GALLON** of water daily. Log the frequency and quality of your bowel movements.

Are you still regular? Have the bowel movements decreased in frequency? Increased? **By day six of juice fasting, it is possible that your trips to the toilet will be less frequent.** When you **DO** have a bowel movement, <u>do not be alarmed</u> if the stools dare darker than usual, almost black. That is **GOOD**. Your body is ridding itself of some very toxic and disease- causing debris! **If you have been constipated, then that reinforces the need for more water.** Did you call your **DESIGNATE** buddy and get active in a forum? I hope you did. The time for procrastination, second-guessing and doubting is over. Now is the time to believe, even if the mind tells you that all of this is poppycock. **We take action anyways.... <u>in spite of ourselves</u>**.

If you are running out of juice again, then it is time to repeat the process you followed on day three. Please do not wait until the last moment to make more juice. And do not lose sight of how much you have left of the other supplies that you need: green tea, seltzer etc. Promptly take stock of your supplies, identify what you may need from the store and go with your friend.

You should definitely **NOT** go to the supermarket alone at this point. If it cannot be helped (*because no friends are available*), then the best way to do it is to blindly walk directly to the items that you need and promptly walk out. Do not linger in the store for any reason. You know how to prepare the juice now. You are becoming a real pro. I am proud of you!

Say to yourself: "*Just for today, I will revisit my journal entries from the last five days. I will ask the God of my understanding for strength to reach my goals and objectives. I am grateful for all I have learned and look forward to the rich blessings that fasting gives my mind, body and spirit. Just for today, I will have joy and happiness - realizing that the best days of my life lie ahead*".

Day 7

Good morning my dear friend: Congratulations. You are reaching the completion of an entire week of fasting! Great job, great job, great job... you are showing amazing resolve and power of decision. You are actually in the minority. Of the billions and billions of human beings on the phase of the earth, very few have accomplished seven full days of voluntary fasting. So I want you to pause for a moment, go stand in front of a mirror and pat yourself on the back saying: "You've done well. I am proud of you and I believe in you."

Go, do that now ... great! Most of us are very quick to chastise ourselves when we fall short, but rarely pause to complement when we reach a goal. I want you to realize the immensity of what you are doing and give yourself the credit that you deserve! Fasting is never easy. Yet you are still here. Well done!!! Now let us buckle down and continue the journey. By **DAY SEVEN** most people are feeling better and better, although weakness and dizziness can be strong. As I have already said, be careful - move slowly, do not rise too quickly from a sitting position.

In rare cases, some people experience fainting. The best way to prevent this is to get as much rest as possible. If you need to go somewhere, ask a friend or family member to drive you. Tread with much, much caution today. Rest, rest and more rest is recommended.

Again, if you are still experiencing strong hunger pangs and/or detox symptoms, just relax. As I mentioned before, green tea helps a lot to soothe symptoms and to give you a pep of energy. Use it as your shield. The same goes with seltzer water. But please make sure not to drink more than four bottles of seltzer water daily as it may irritate your stomach and cause more discomfort.

Are you spending time in the journal and reaching out to your **DESIGNATE** buddy? Do not ignore or set aside this recommendation. It is very important to have somebody close to you who knows what you are doing and is in your corner. A 15-minute chat with a close friend who supports you will go a long ways in renewing your strength and allowing a wave of hunger to pass. We are going forward and making progress. But we have to remain very vigilant, as the mind is a cunning foe.

As always, drink as much water as possible during the day. Spend some time writing about what you are feeling physically and mentally, as well as any other insight, thoughts and/or ideas that may come your way. Writing on the journal constantly while fasting is (*by far*) one of the best ways to make it through those rough spots.

Remember: each moment of fasting awakens your spiritual side more and more... none of this that you are going through will be in vain. Keep your eyes on the prize; keep reminding yourself of your objective and do not let the mind focus your attention **ONLY** on "*how uncomfortable I feel*".

You can do it! Keep at it and do **<u>NOT</u>** give up!

Say to yourself: *"Today I will remember my goals and not focus only on the discomfort. I will emphasize the huge positive health benefits that I am receiving through fasting. I will keep the vision of that "new me" on my mind. I will walk through whatever challenge comes my way. I thank the God of my understanding for the strength, grace and power to make it through these 24 hours of fasting".*

Day 8

Good morning: Congratulations on making it to another day. You are moving deeper and deeper into your land of miracles. How are you feeling? Are you sleeping well? Remember that you have the chamomile tea, tryptophan and valerian root to help settle you down at night so that you can sleep. If you find yourself feeling agitated during the day, take a tryptophan tablet and have a cup of chamomile tea. It will help to center you and give you breathing room to get through the immediate challenge. How's the juice drinking coming along?

Two large glasses of water upon awakening, your first eight-to-twelve-ounce glass of juice one hour later, and more juice every four hours... maximum 64 ounces per day. You may be running low on juice again. By this point, juicing is probably a walk in the park, right? How is that going? If you feel comfortable, you may wish to experiment with the fruit and veggie charts that I showed you earlier so that you can play around with the taste of the juice. There's still plenty of time, however. If you are unsure, then just stick to the basic recipe for now.

Today I want to start sharing with you a system that helps me a lot whenever I am fasting. **How To R.E.A.C.H. My Goals**. I use the acronym R.E.A.C.H. to illustrate these 5 steps because that's your job as a juice fasting practitioner ... **to reach and achieve the weight loss and health-improvement goals that you want. .**

To bring to reality the changes that will allow you to have the quality of life that you want. Is that not what you want? I am sure that it is. Here is how R.E.A.C.H expands:

R – **RELEASE** yourself from guilt and self-condemnation.
E – **ENJOY** life today -right here, right now.
A – **AVOID** sugar, starches, caffeine, fats & junk food of any kind.
C – **CONSIDER** the impact of what you are doing.
H – **HANG** on to your dreams and never back down.

There is a lot of power in those five points. Let's begin to look at them one by one.

Step 1: "R" RELEASE Yourself from Guilt & Self-Condemnation: On speaking to more than 50 people who started a long-term fast and failed - guess what the number one reason was for their fall? Yep -> Guilt and Self-Condemnation. *"I just did not feel I was worth all of this trouble,"* said Jim, 47, who has been 80 pounds overweight for five years and struggles with hypertension. *"I have always messed up. I have never done anything right when it comes to food. I had faith in failure; I did not believe I could lose the weight. All I constantly did was put myself down; I just couldn't stand the sight of myself,"* he said.

Sadly, this describes the mentality of many people that e-mail me. Can you relate? In which way do you find yourself caught in guilt and self-condemnation? Write about it in the journal.

Get to know that voice that wants to bring you down, that wants to keep you from accomplishing your goals. When I get these emails, I always ask very important question: What mistakes have you made that you keep putting yourself down for? Answer that question in the journal to see what comes out.

If you have tried fasting and/or dieting in the past and have failed, then it is highly probable that you say negative things to yourself related to those unsuccessful attempts. It is possible that being lean and healthy is a far-fetched ideal that, in your mind, you do not feel you deserve or are good enough to attain. Whatever the situation might have been ... whatever failures you may have had in the past ... no matter how many times you have tried it before and failed ... TODAY IS A BRAND NEW DAY! Let the past go!

"Visualize yourself dropping a box filled with the past into a bottomless pit. Gone! Forgive yourself for your mistakes! Continuously rehashing past mistakes will **NEVER** produce the positive change we are after in this course." One can fast for a hundred days. But the change will be fleeting if destructive mental patterns are not challenged. You already have started to confront the negativity.

It is imperative that you rid yourself of guilt and self-condemnation. If your mind is full of *"what could have been but never was"* or *"what I have done to myself"* or *"the worthless or inferior person that I am,"* *(or any number of variations of this negativity)*

– then you will **ALWAYS** find some reason to break the fast. The mind will usually feed you some negativity like: *"why should I deserve to accomplish something that will make my life better?"*

Step 2 "E" ENVISION Yourself at the Ideal Weight / Health: Another top reason why persons start a long-term fast and then break it prematurely is because *"they allow the mental negativity and detox symptoms to cloud their vision of what they want to accomplish."* An effective way to sidestep this common pitfall is to create a collage of body pictures that are in line with your goals and spend time daily looking at them – especially when you are fasting and struggling with hunger and/or detox symptoms. You told me that you were willing to do whatever it takes. So today I am going to take you at your word and ask you to do a little project. "

Do this:

Browse through magazines and cut out pictures of sleek and fit bodies. **Note**: You can, of course, also do this by surfing the web and printing out the images. Cut the head out of a picture of yourself from some family album or other photograph. Paste it to the body picture image from the magazine. This worked immensely for me. Looking at my face in the thin body from the magazine kept me focused on what I wanted to accomplish. **Looking at that photo interrupted the negativity that urged me to give in**. It helped to snap away from the trap and press forward with my goals!"

Paste the pictures in *"trigger"* locations such as the bathroom mirror, the nightstand or desk right next to your bed (*so it is the last thing you see at night and the first image you intake upon awakening*), and - *of course* – the refrigerator door. Every morning when you get up look at it and tell yourself: **"This is me. This is how I want to look physically. I can do this."** **Remember; nothing tastes as good as thin feels!** Build a *"collage"* of fit bodies taking part in a variety of athletic and recreational activities and stick your head into the bodies. This *"envision"* step is a mighty weapon that you can place in your fasting arsenal. It is truly amazing. I realize that, for many, this whole thing about building a collage, pasting their face on fit bodies etc may seem like to totally cheesy and stupid practice that cannot possibly yield anything positive. There's that voice again... talking down about the things that are given to you to help you. Ignore the voice, ignore *'feeling silly'* and do the exercise anyway. Trust me... it will help you a lot. You still have a ways to go and need all of the weapons that you can get. So get to work on the collage and we will continue with step 3 tomorrow.

Say to yourself: *"Today I am releasing all negativity and resistance. I becoming willing to completely let go of all thoughts that want to discourage me and cause me to fail. There is no failure for me today because I release all of it from my mind. I let it go completely and watch it as it leaves my life for good. Instead, today I am filled with passion, strength, commitment and determination. I cannot be moved because the Grace and peace of God is upon me...*

I am safe to continue in my path. And I can rejoice because, today... all is well."

Day 9

Good morning my dear brother / sister. How are you feeling today? You are almost at double digits. That's the point of no return, you know? You are moving further and further into the process. Can there possibly be anything that could cause you to give up at this point? No way! You are locked in my friend. You are totally committed. You drew a line in the sand and separated the past from the future. And it is in this present that your new future is being created. By being willing to continue through this fasting path, and by facing the challenge, your entire destiny is being rewritten from inside your heart OUT to your body and the world.

Today is likely time to juice again. By now you should feel pretty comfortable with the process. I know that I did. Initially I hated it, but it grew on me. I understood that prepping the fruits and veggies, juicing and bottling the juice are all acts of love that I am giving to myself. And so it is with you. What you are doing is the true meaning of self-love.

Being willing to walk through discomfort and do things that you normally may not have done, all for the purpose of helping to improve your health. If a friend did all of that for you, would you not consider him or her special? Yes, of course.

The relationship with yourself, the most important of all, is also healing. The more you move forward and stay the course, the more you show to that man or woman in the mirror that you care for him or her. Let's continue to step 3 of the acronym R.E.A.C.H.

Step 3 "A" AVOID Sugar, Starches, Caffeine, Fats & All Junk Food. We have touched on this before; the need to make a firm decision that **NO LONGER** will you allow these foods to control you, harm your health and cause you to become overweight. No longer! Make a commitment with yourself RIGHT **HERE AND RIGHT NOW** that, once the fast is over, you will **NOT** return to these toxic and destructive foods. They were part of the past. However, they no longer serve any purpose in your life. You are aware of their allure and destructive power and are **NO LONGER** willing to give in to their subtle invitations. No more, no more, no more... that filth is **OUT** of your life for good. Of course, the implementation of this decision you are making is done 'one day at a time.' Each day, when I wake up, I pray and ask the God of my understanding to help keep me away from that first bite of the junk foods that used to harm me. If I don't take the first bite, then I cannot binge and fall by the wayside. Today, I pass on this same willingness to you... will you take it?

Step 4 "C" CONSIDER the Impact of What You are Doing. This step challenges you to expand your fasting journal... to stop skimping on the surface and, instead, go deep into your heart and identify the impact of what you are doing. What have you been writing about in your journal? Have you written at all? Or have you scribbled a few "*quick thoughts*" without giving it any profound thought?

I hope that has **NOT** been the case. If it has, then I want to give you a subtle nudge and ask you to do it! **NOW** is the time to grasp this assignment and start to really dig into it with everything that you have! I have NEVER seen anybody complete a long-term fast that did not have clear, written reasons as to why they were doing it. Step 2 helps you to reinforce what you want to accomplish, visually. **This fourth step, however, is the most crucial of all because, with it, you are exploring your soul's deepest and fondest dreams.** You are digging into the very core of your existence to determine what you consider to be your heart-felt goals and ideals as these relate to health.

"*Your dreams, hopes and ambitions must all be in writing so that you can see and read them.*" Why? Because most "fasters" suffer from a very short memory, especially when amidst a long-term fast and stricken by hunger pains and detox symptoms. They seem to forget the heartbreak and devastation of even a week ago. How they felt when on their last binge of overeating; when they looked at themselves in the mirror and saw the rolls of flab all over. The disgust and remorse of the past is forgotten. The mind, as usual, will attempt to "*trap you in time*" by erasing your long-term goals from memory. **It will persuade you to give up.**

If you have nothing in writing that you can go to and remind yourself why you are doing what you are doing, then you'll be very vulnerable to the mind's subterfuges. This baffling mental assault caused me to fall many, many times.

Permanent change requires focused and consistent action. I will give you every weapon in the arsenal. But if you file the information and allow it to collect dust, then it will not do much good. You may not be prepared for the battle and could become a casualty. We have had enough of that, haven't we? Today, spend more time writing the *'reasons'* why you are doing this fast. Add detail... **heart-felt emotion and detail**. Spill your heart into the paper and hold nothing back.

We are not doing this to be martyrs or masochists. Rather, we are doing it to improve the quality of our lives. <u>**In short**</u>: **The words written in your journal <u>ALONG</u> with the visual stimulus from the Step 2 collage create a potent "two-punch" combination that will help you tremendously to counteract detox symptoms, hunger and negativity.**

Day 10

You have broken into phase two of your juice fast. Ten days is a **HUGE** accomplishment. Of the dozens and dozens of people that I have coached in the past five years, hardly any make it to ten days of fasting. They want to fast. They are honestly struggling and know they need to lose weight. But, for some reason, they are unable to muster the inner strength and determination to make it very far.

So you, my friend, are an amazing person. I wish I could be there where you are so that I can literally huge you and tell you how proud I am of you. I mean it. We are together in this journey. Your breakthrough is my breakthrough because we are fellow travelers in the road of self-mastery. Isn't that what fasting is? Self-mastery? Yes. **And you are moving further and further into a powerful chasm of self-realization that will lead you to all of your dreams.** Keep going!

Step 5 "H" HANG on To Your Dreams and NEVER Back Down! This step won't work unless you have done steps two and four. Here is where you are able to see why you are taking time from your life to do this fast and produce these changes in your life.

Join me in a quick journey through time, space, the past, the present and future. Let us go deep into our hearts and minds and find the strength to overcome.

Maybe you have tried it all before and have always gained the weight back. Perhaps you have tried every diet under the sun and nothing has worked. Maybe you are ill ...

...maybe you have very little hope that anything will ever work. But, then, when you start to write about your dreams and goals ... something happens inside of you. For a minute, even for just an instant, you start to believe that... maybe; just maybe... it is possible. You visualize yourself wearing that dress or pant-size that you always dreamed of. You think of wearing a bathing suit and feeling good about walking around on the beach ... proud of what you have accomplished...

... You no longer have to be ashamed or hide from the world. Or maybe you dream of a day when you will not feel sluggish and full of inertia and apathy towards life. You want to go up a flight of stairs without huffing and puffing ...

...you want to think clearly and be rid of the confusion and overall mental fatigue that plagues you. You want to look and feel better ... you want your life to be full of energy and health. You want to walk this earth and be the best that you possibly can ...

... you want to maximize your time here and give your family, your community and the world the very best of you... no matter what your role in life may be ... whether you are a parent, an employee, a manager, a director or an international mogul...

you need your health, right? You want your world to be filled with optimism and hope

... So that when all is said and done you can, in your heart of hearts, have absolutely no regrets. You gave it your very best and had the courage to overcome your struggles. And the struggles themselves served to forge your character so that you could positively-influence the lives of everyone around you ...

... Amazing, huh? How the very struggle that was there to bring us down eventually became our greatest asset ...

...These are many of the elements that make up life... that make up destiny and fate. And they are all in your hands – right here, right now. The fork in the road is before you. The two paths are clearly made and in your sights. Which will it be? Will you give up and continue to go through life thinking about *"what could have been?"* Or are you going to press on and reach the goals?

...Put the past behind you. Forget about all of your failures and disappointments. We have all had them. Today marks a brand new beginning. The slate is clean and the sky is the limit. This is the first day of the rest of your life...

...Believe ... believe, my friend, that you are worth it. Believe that you can reach **ALL** of your dreams and goals.

Do not allow your mind, people or the world tell you – even for a minute – that you are finished or that you are not strong enough to make it...

...They are lies, lies ... all lies! **YOU CAN MAKE IT!** And you are sooo worth it! This is the moment of truth ... the moment where a brand new destiny is being written for you by the universe...

... And you are now walking the road-less-traveled of **CHANGE** that will take you where you always dreamed... there are no more limits... no more impossibilities. You are free!"

Day 11

You are now on day 11, one step closer to the goal. Have you weighed yourself? How much weight have you lost? The goal is 30 pounds, but - as I said before - you very well could lose even more. It all depends on how your body responds. This is the final motivational message. However, there is plenty of 'meat' in all of them to keep you going until the end of the fast. Please return to the message from day 1 tomorrow and make your way through them once again. Apply the suggestions that I give you with greater emphasis this time around. Whatever you may have skipped the first time around, now you have the opportunity to do it again.

This is what I call "**The Next Phase of Development**." This basically represents the rest of your life. The collection of 24-hours that will depict your existence from today forward. Which way will it go? Will you persist with the principles you have learned and accomplish/retain your freedom? What will determine what the coming years will be like for you? That's what this fast is all about. My message to you today is this: **FREEDOM CARRIES SACRIFICE**. This is particularly true when it comes to weight loss, body cleansing and changing eating habits. I am sure that by this point you know exactly what I'm talking about. Hunger and detox symptoms are always looming and beckoning you to give up. At least that is the case with me. I am not "*cured*." For the past ten years I have not relapsed into binging.

I have successfully kept myself at a trim 200 pounds. But I have had to sacrifice. I don't mean sacrifice in a morbid or ascetic way. What I mean is that I have had to realize that, if I wanted to protect my weight and health, I had to realize that I was not *"just like everyone else."* The crowd eats mindlessly and pays little or no attention to future health consequences. The crowd wants - the crowd eats. The crowd craves - the crowd gives in. That is the status quo and the way in which millions live their lives. But that is **NOT** what you have learned here. You must separate yourself from *"the crowd"* and treat yourself with the unique respect and delicate-kindness that you deserve. Your choices in food from now on can **NEVER** be the same. **You have awakened from your slumber and can no longer be counted in the sleeping masses**. You want to be lean, healthy and vibrant. And it is your desire to accomplish/maintain this not *"just for a little while,"* but for life - right? Yes, it is!

Say to yourself: *"Today I surrender completely to this fast, mind, body and spirit. I open my heart and mind to receive the strength and power of God, which fills me with infinite power, wisdom and supernatural determination. Nothing can stop me because I have let go of all the negative. I may hear it and feel it, but I no longer react to it. All negativity MUST yield to my spiritual determination. I believe that the light of God inside of me burns through all negativity and destroys every behavior, habit or belief system that leads me away from my goals.*
I am renewed in mind, body and spirit and am filled with peace. All is well. I am loved. I'm safe and free!"

Chapter 21
Ending the Fast

Breaking a fast is the most important part of the process, right? Yes, I've said that to you like four times already. I'm sure you're sick of hearing me say it. But it is absolutely true. I have run into many people who fast for thirty days and more... but they break it inappropriately. This is unwise and dangerous. The digestive system has been inactive, so we have to wake it up slowly and steadily. You can literally place your life in danger if you do not break a fast adequately.

One man that wrote me said he fasted for 14 days and broke it with a cheeseburger. He got horribly ill and his stomach swelled up like a balloon. He nearly ruptured his stomach lining and died. I was heartbroken for him. Well intentioned... but not properly informed. So we must tread carefully. Not only that, but I also want you to come face-to-face with hunger and **NOT** give in to it. **Hunger comes back strong when one first breaks a fast**. The key is to stick to the schedule I have outlined.

Do not "*hurry*" things because you "*think*" that you are ready. I have fallen prey to that mental trickery and can tell you that it is **NO FUN**. It takes hard work to complete a 30-day fast. There is nothing more discouraging than to give away the benefits at the last moment. **That is like the man whose boat sinks and he is forced to swim for days in the cold, dark ocean.**

Finally, he sees the beach up ahead but, just as he is about to touch land, he decides to stop swimming and sink to the bottom. What! All of what swimming for nothing? No way!

Here's my point: The stricter you are with the process of breaking a fast, the greater the benefits and the stronger your foundation will be for long-term success. And <u>LONG TERM</u> success is what we want, right? Right!

Post Fast Shopping List

On the last 48 hours of the fast, go to the market and pick up some supplies. We'll need some fresh produce. Here's my personal "breaking a fast" fruit/veggie combination: apples, pears, oranges, celery, carrots, spinach and watercress. Your body will receive a tremendous jolt of nutrition. Of course if you have a personal juicing recipe, go ahead and use it.

But make sure that you combine <u>BOTH</u> fruits and vegetables. Set aside several apples and pears for eating only. If you prefer, you can use cantaloupe, apricots and/or papaya. Stay away from overly-sweet fruit like honeydew. Don't juice them. We will need them as part of the re-feeding process. Also from the produce section, get some lettuce, tomatoes, cucumbers and a couple of lemons. In addition to the produce, you'll need a bottle of **Probiotics** to help repopulate the "*good bacteria*" in your stomach. Check in the dairy section to see if you find **Kefir.**

Unlike yogurt which contains transient bacteria that do not repopulate the digestive tract, Kefir has active, growing and "living bacteria". This is a marvelous boost to your system, and will swiftly repopulate the digestive tract. Moreover, get some chicken broth packets, some low-fat milk, a bag of flax seeds, a small bottle of olive oil and a package of some good oat bran cereal (*not the sugar-filled commercial type please!*). These items can usually be found at the health-food section of many supermarkets. If not, then you can order them online. Finally, purchase a bottle of some natural juice. I use grape and orange, but you can choose whatever type you like best, even vegetable juice. Keep it simple. A good juice from the health-food section in your local supermarket will more than suffice. After day three you will be juicing a combination of fruit and vegetable juice. But for starters, a good bottled **NATURAL JUICE** is enough. That is the end of the shopping list! Please make sure to have all of these items in place by Day 30. Do not wait until the last moment. For guidance, here is a shopping list with the post-fast supplies that you will need:

1 Bottle of Probiotics: Probiotics help to repopulate the "*good bacteria*" in your stomach, a great deal of which is expelled during a long-term fast.

1 Bottle of Kefir: Check in the dairy section of your local supermarket and see if you see Kefir there. Unlike yogurt which contains transient bacteria that do not repopulate the digestive tract, Kefir has active, growing and "*living bacteria*". This is a marvelous boost to your system, and will swiftly repopulate the digestive tract.

3-5 Chicken Broth Packets

1 Jug of Non-Fat Milk

1 Bag of Flax Seeds

1 Bottle of Olive Oil

1 Box Oat Bran Cereal (*not the sugar-filled commercial type please*!).

1 Bottle Natural Juice (Fruit & Veggie Mixtures Are Best)

Chapter 22
How to Break the Fast

If you reading this page, then it means that you completed the 30-day fast and are now prepared to enter re-feeding. I could just kiss you. You are awesome. **NOW**, we must press forward with great caution and start to break the fast. Since you have been drinking lots of fruit and veggie juice *(as well as pulp)*, breaking this fast will be very simple. Let's get to it!

Post-Fast Day 1

For breakfast, cut up an apple or pear in four slices and sit down to eat.

Eat each half **VERY** slowly and chew it until it dissolves in your mouth. Resist the desire to eat quickly. Chew each piece of fruit at least 20 times prior to swallowing. Count each chew. **DONT CHEAT**! Spend at least TWO minutes chewing and swallowing each of the four pieces of fruit. That means that you should spend roughly **TEN** minutes eating your "*meal*". To wash down the fruit, drink a 12-ounce glass of 50-percent water & 50-percent juice. We just gave the body some solids for the first time in a while. **It is best to water down the juice and be cautiou**s. Take **ONE** capsule of Probiotics. Wait **FOUR** hours. Once the time has passed, repeat the breakfast meal with another piece of fruit and another watered-down glass of juice. Wait another **FOUR** hours.

Have a **THIRD** fruit/juice meal. Mix the fruits. You can, for example, have an apple in the morning and pears in the afternoon and evening. Steer clear of citrus (*you can drink orange juice but hold off on EATING oranges*). Stick to apples and pears for now. Go to bed. Eat **NOTHING** else. Stay away from the kitchen!

Post-Fast Day 2

On the second day of breaking the fast, repeat the **EXACT SAME** process as yesterday for breakfast and lunch. Don't forget to take **ONE** capsule of probiotics. An apple or pear in the morning (*or whatever fruit you chose*), apple or pear in the afternoon and apple or pear in the evening. Each meal washed down with a 12-ounce glass of watered-down fruit/veggie juice. **Watch your thoughts and emotions very carefully**. The mind will attempt to trick you into eating a full-course meal.

You may find yourself rationalizing "*why it's ok*" to eat this, eat that ... etc. **RESIST**! The digestive system is shifting back from feeding solely on stored fat to relying (*again*) on the daily consumption of food. You may experience a more substantial bowel movement today. But you must be careful and follow the directions. The wrong meal now and a lot of the work you have done can be ruined. You need to take it very slowly and walk around as if on eggshells for a few days. In the evening, at your usual dinner time, have a cup of chicken broth. Use one envelope only as broth has a lot of sodium.

Post-Fast Day 3

If your stomach is feeling fine and there is no pain or discomfort, then today you can introduce salad sprinkled with flax seeds (*one or two tablespoons*). Flax seeds are very good for digestion and will help your digestive system as you re-introduce solid foods. Eat an apple in the morning with juice **AND** have a medium-sized plate of lettuce, cucumbers and baby tomatoes for lunch. **NO DRESSING OR SALT**! You can get away with a tiny "*sprinkle*" of olive oil and vinegar... but that is all. Do not go overboard on the salad. Keep quantities small. **TIP**: Go to the supermarket and purchase several pre-made salad kits. As always, do not forget to take your Probiotics in the morning with breakfast.

Choose the "*simple*" kits, which usually include lettuce, carrots, cabbage and the like ... **NOTHING MORE**. We're looking for a basic "*bare bones*" salad at this point. Eat **HALF** a bag per meal. That way you take away the need of having to prepare a salad and hang out in the kitchen. Half a bag of a pre-made salad kit is more than enough for starters. If the kit you purchased comes with dressing and croutons, **DISCARD THEM**! Add food types and amounts slowly.

When it comes to breaking a fast, **SLOW IS FAST**. What I mean by that is this: If you are thorough, cautious and meticulous from start to finish (*without rushing*), then chances are pretty good that you will **NOT** have to repeat the process.

Going through the sacrifice of a long-term fast only to gain the weight back later is truly heartbreaking. The time is **NOW** for you to start mastering your appetites and learning that *"just because the body says it wants it, does NOT mean you have to give in to it."*

If a little baby got angry because you took away a butcher's knife he was playing with - would you feel bad about it? Would you feel guilty when the baby started crying and throwing a tantrum? Of course not. The same is with the stomach and our appetites. They **MUST** be disciplined - sometimes forcefully. Have another salad for lunch along with an apple or pear and some juice (*you don't have to water it down anymore if your body is responding well*). For dinner, you can add a **SMALL** plate of steamed vegetables <u>WITHOUT</u> butter.

I like broccoli, carrots, squash and cauliflower. You can sprinkle a tiny dab of olive oil for taste. Add flax seeds on top. Make sure to drink lots of water - **at least half-a-gallon daily**. All in all, today you have given your body salads and vegetables **IN ADDITION** to the fruit and juices. If at any time you start to feel stomach discomfort, add another 24 hours of just juices and fruit. When breaking a fast, always step <u>BACK</u> at least <u>ONE</u> day if you feel your body needs more time. Listen to what your body is <u>REALLY</u> telling you. Don't make a decision based on hunger! Rather, close your eyes, go past the hunger and listen to what the body is saying. Is the digestive system processing the fruit, salad and vegetables properly?

Are you having trouble having a bowel movement? If you are straining to pass stool, then you are forcing the body to process way too much food, too soon. Slow down if you are in doubt. Again I repeat: **SLOW IS FAST**!

Post-Fast Day 4 and Beyond

On Day 4, you can start to eat small pieces of lean poultry. You can steam-cook a breast of chicken very nicely on a pan with its own juices, a little water and a tiny sprinkle of olive oil. Be very light on the salt when seasoning. If you have a broiler, then go ahead and use it. This piece of meat is not intended to be a *"gourmet"* experience. In fact, it should be pretty bland. You are eating it **NOT** as a *"fine-dining"* experience, but rather to continue awakening the digestive system.

And very important: Chew slowly! Resist the urge to gorge at all times. **For dinner, try this**: A small chicken breast with a salad and **HALF** a baked potato **WITHOUT** butter. One cup of brown rice is also a good choice. I like the boil-in-the-bag rice because it cooks quickly and actually tastes decent. Sprinkle a dash of parmesan cheese on the potato for taste. The key at this phase of breaking a fast is to keep the portions small. **If, after you eat a meal on day 4, you start to have stomach aches, then you know you ate too much or you added some spice that was not permitted.** Beyond Day 4, continue to eat the **SAME** foods I have just described. You can exchange chicken for fish (*Tilapia and Grouper are my personal favorites*).

You also can eat different fruits according to your taste. If you eat red meat, I strongly encourage you to **NOT** eat any for at least **ONE** month after breaking a fast. Your body is clean! **This is a great time for you to take some serious stock of where you have been, where you are and where you want to go**. If you look back and realize that you **DO NOT** want to return to the way you were, then - *as I said earlier* - the **TIME IS NOW** to make some definite lifestyle changes and pay whatever price you have to pay for the sake of your health.

Weight Gain After Fasting

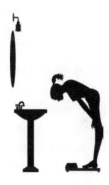

No matter how closely you observe the re-feeding regimen, breaking a fast always leads to weight gain of 5-10 pounds in the first 14 to 21 days. This is no reason to freak out, as many do. The weight gain is a totally normal reaction to a long-term fast. The body was in ketosis for a long time. This is basically the body's starvation/survival mode. During the fast, the body scavenged the body in search of anything it could devour - eating pure fat on a daily basis.

When you break the fast, the body, still alarmed from the fast, begins to 'hoard' energy *'just in case'* another survival situation happens (**the body doesn't know that you were fasting intentionally**). In addition, while fasting the metabolism slows down considerably. When you couple the body's exit from starvation mode and a sluggish metabolism, the result is the weight gain I've described. <u>**AND**</u>, we cannot forget that at the point of breaking a fast there will also be a certain amount of water weight gain. All of this is normal. There is no reason to be upset. What matters is that you continue to eat a clean diet with portion control. Over the following weeks, if you keep eating clean and healthy, then you will find that you are starting to lose the initial weight that was gained. Fasting produces very fast weight loss. That means that, after fasting, your body size is likely quite smaller than it was when you began. The body needs time to get used to this new order of things. Don't obsess on scales and numbers. Instead, go to the nearest sports shop and purchase a device to measure body fat. Rather than the scale, start to rely more and more on your body fat level.

That will give you a much more precise verdict of where you are. I had times when the scale said I weighed four pounds more, but my body fat levels had actually decreased! As you can see, pounds can be deceiving. But body fat measurements don't lie and are always constant. Plus, scales cause many of us to get way too emotional. And that often leads to discouragement and the 'screw it' syndrome. You have come way too far to succumb to this.

Chapter 23
The Next Step

I would love to be there to rejoice with you and see how much weight you lost, and how you are feeling. Feel free to come to **FitnessThroughFasting.com** and drop me a line through the *'contact us'* link with comments. I would very much like to hear how the fast went and what your comments are about the way I presented the material. Seriously, congratulations on this wonderful achievement.

Now you need to establish a new order of things. I encourage you to **<u>IMMEDIATELY</u>** find a meal structure that you can adopt permanently and follow in perpetuity I encourage you to read my other book **"The Permanent Weight Loss Diet)** where I outline a detailed and aggressive eating plan that I believe can help you go the distance. Meanwhile, work at staying away from these foods:

Post Fasting Banned Foods

*Enriched Flour
*Salt
* Sugar
* Fried Foods
* Cheese
* Dairy Products
* Red Meat
* Alcohol (an occasional glass of wine or drink is fine)

* **Butter or Margarine**
* **Fruit Juices**
* **Regular Ketchup (except low sodium)**
*Junk Food of ANY Kind**

Do this alone and you will be on your way to keeping the weight off. You need a structured meal plan... period. The sooner you can start with that, the stronger the foundation you will have for long-term weight loss.

Chapter 24
Motivation

Over the past few days, I've been working on a Motivation page for the main **Fitness Through Fasting**.com website. I want to share some of the content with you in hopes that, if you have been struggling, this message may help to *"refill your tank"* and push you to keep going. **Here goes:**

What is motivation? Why is it so important, and how is it regained when lost? These are very important questions. Motivation is a *"feeling"* that inspires us to accomplish our goals; be they a business project, raising children, helping others or – *as in our case* – weight loss and health improvement. The dictionary defines motivation as; *"A feeling of enthusiasm, interest, or commitment that makes somebody want to do something."*

This enthusiasm, however, is threatened on a daily basis by many pressures and situations. As our lives become increasingly complicated with work, finances, social pressure, health issues and/or family relations (*among others*), we can start to feel overwhelmed, drained, tired and unhealthy. Our energy is depleted and we become discouraged. At this point comes the desire to *"give up"*. Negative thoughts emerge like: *"I can't do this... this is too hard"* or *"there's no solution to this problem... what's the use anyways"*. We start to *"lack motivation"* when we lose mental focus of our goals and ideals.

When this happens, the result can be depression, hopelessness and immobilization. I've been there enough times to know exactly just how painful this state of *"unmotivation"* can be. Lack of motivation drains our capacity to take action. Stagnation sets in. **Our sense of purpose is zapped.**

We stop doing the very things we need to do to triumph over circumstances. We become trapped in a prison of negativity and emotional pain within our own minds. Realizing <u>THAT</u> is actually the way out, I have found. Whenever we feel drained and lacking motivation, we must immediately become conscious that the problem is <u>NOT</u> with any external situation per se, but rather with our thoughts and perceptions of what is happening around us.

Recovering motivation is **<u>SIMPLER</u>** than one may think. We need to take things **ONE DAY AT A TIME**; stop allowing external pressures to overwhelm and deplete our energy. Most of all, realize that <u>NOW</u> is all that any of us ever have. The past and future do not exist and are, in the end, <u>just an illusion</u>. Return to the present in your heart, mind and spirit. Realize that at *"this moment in time"* everything is as it should be. **You are lacking nothing**.

Stop trying to accomplish and solve everything at once. Life is far too short to become besieged by an avalanche of external demands. Focus <u>ONLY</u> on what is in front of you (*look at your feet; can you be anywhere else but where you are?*).

Trust that each situation will eventually be resolved in the measure that you remain centered and do not allow yourself to become overwhelmed.

To stay inspired, to retain self-motivation, **we must first take care of ourselves**. Stop and smell the roses on the way to work, take a moment to breathe-in the sweet scent of life, love and laughter. We need to value the "*who*" of what we are <u>NOW</u> - in this moment in time.

The more we learn to accept who we are exactly as we are right here and right now, the faster we will reopen the door to the TRUE spirit of motivation. To stay inspired and motivated, we must also learn to give to others. Whatever you do to motivate, cheer and uplift another will come back to you 110% and fill you with the light, energy, strength and motivation that you need to transcend challenges and reach your highest potential.

See You In The Next Volume!
God bless,

ROBERT DAVE JOHNSTON

Grab The Entire Collection:

Volume 1: The 'Permanent Weight Loss' Diet

Volume 2: The Intermittent Fasting Weight Loss Formula

Volume 3: How to Lose 30 Pounds (Or More) In 30 Days With Juice Fasting

Volume 4: Lose The Belly Fat Fast, And For Good!

Volume 5: Lose the Emotional Baggage: Transform Your Mind & Spirit With Fasting

Volume 6: How to Break a Fast (or Diet) and Keep The Weight Off

Volume 7: Compilation Volumes 1-6 -> Get All 5 For The Price Of 3!

Also by Robert Dave Johnston:

How To Lose Weight & Keep it Off By Transforming The Mind & Behaviors

Volume 1: How to Build a Rock-Solid Foundation That Supports Long-Term Weight Loss

Volume 2: How To Lose Weight & Keep it Off By Reprogramming The Subconscious Mind

Volume 3: How To Beat Diet Hunger and Junk Food Cravings

Volume 4: How to Escape the Diet "Time Trap" and Succeed in Weight Loss

Volume 5: How To Cheat On Your Diet (And Get Away With It)

Volume 6, Compilation: Get all 5 For The Price Of 3

Also By Robert Dave Johnston:

Detoxify Your Body, Lose Weight, Get Healthy & Transform Your Life

Volume 1- The 10-Day 'At Home' Colon Cleansing Formula

Volume 2- The 30-Day Kidney, Parasite & Liver Detox Weight Loss Method

Volume 3- Lose Weight Fast & Detoxify With Intermittent Fasting & At-Home Coffee Enemas

Volume 4 - Compilation: Get All 4 For The Price Of 2! Detoxify Your Body, Lose Weight, Get Healthy & Transform Your Life - Volumes 1-3 [

Don't forget to check the articles and growing health community at: FitnessThroughFasting.com

7371912R00081

Made in the USA
San Bernardino, CA
03 January 2014